Anti-Inflammatory Diet Cookbook

Healthy and Delicious Recipes to Reduce Inflammation Naturally and Boost Your Immune System

By Susan Kellery

Table of Contents

Introduction

As with any problem, nature seems to give us simple ways to solve it. We've heard recently in the news about how inflammation can affect the body. Numerous disorders have been linked to inflammation, including Alzheimer's, kidney disease, Crohn's disease, Parkinson's, asthma, respiratory disease, breast cancer, high cholesterol, heart disease, hypoglycemia, degenerative arthritis, colon cancer, rheumatoid arthritis, uterine cancer, tuberculosis, and osteoporosis.

The mechanism will be referred to as inflammation for those of you who have sprained your ankle and seen the accompanying swelling, warmth, and pains. But does the general public or the fitness instructors really grasp this disease process in depth? Inflammation is a prevalent part of our lexicon, we read about it in newspapers and blogs, and hear it on TV.

Merely putting the inflammation is a non-specific response to cell injury. Injury can be caused by trauma, infection, or autoimmune reactions. White blood cells (WBCs), blood vessels, and chemical mediators are involved in this complex process. The body relies on its own defense on the inflammatory process. Inflammation actually destroys species such as viruses and bacteria in our tissues to prevent their replication and dissemination. It also restricts tissue damage to a finite area and slows out the spread of microbes that enter this. Often responsible for removing debris and making way for the reconstruction of damaged tissues and organs is inflammation. Inflammation can have two components: cellular and vascular. The cellular portion comprises immune cells called neutrophils and monocytes that are responsible for "eating up" the bad guys (viruses, bacteria, etc.) through a process called phagocytosis. Such cells are commonly referred to as phagocytes. They will migrate and adhere to vessel walls at the injury site (a process called marginalization) in the event of acute injury or insult. In a process called emigration, oppressed cells will go through the vessel walls to the exact location of the damage or the diseased tissue. In the case of neutrophils, this can take six to 24 hours, and in the case of monocytes, it may take 24-48 hours. This accounts for the pause we find in the healing phase following an acute insult. At the injury site, the vascular portion is responsible for vasodilatation, increased blood flow, and increased capillary permeability.

The complement system, or which plasma proteins are produced by our bodies to attract WBCs and degranulate mast cells, is yet another component of inflammation. They are classified as C-3, C-5, (as in bradykinin and prostaglandin E) kinins. These chemical mediators are known to cause pain at the injury site, which is responsible for the diseased tissue swell. The arachidonic acid group of plasma proteins produces leukotrienes that control inflammation (PGD2, E2, F2, Thromboxane A2). The thromboxanes and arachidonic acid pathways are blocked by non-steroidal anti-inflammatory medications (NSAID) and steroids (cortisone) to help relieve inflammation. That is why, when an acute insult happens, Aspirin or Motrin is regularly prescribed.

Interferon (alfa, beta, and gamma) and tumor necrosis factor (TNF) are other chemical mediators. Among other things, these chemical mediators are also partially responsible for causing fever. Fever is one of the ways the body has to cope with invasion by viruses and bacteria. It is known that those chemical mediators react to NSAIDs. For this purpose, they are used to battle fevers.

Inflammation findings include leukocytosis (an elevated WBC blood count), lack of appetite, fatigue, rise in our deep sleep time, weight loss, and weakness. With inflammation resolution, we see a return to average vascular permeability, edema lessening, or tissue swelling as plasma proteins are absorbed through the lymphatic system and macrophage phagocytosis removal of damaged cellular debris.

Finding ways to reduce the body's chronic inflammation will lead to a longer, healthier life and lower your risk of contracting certain diseases.

Chapter 1: The Inflammation
What Is Inflammation?

Inflammation is a crucial part of the response to injury and infection provided by the immune system. It is the way the body activates the immune system to heal and repair damaged tissue, and it protects itself against foreign invaders, such as viruses and bacteria.

Wounds will fester without treatment as a physiological response, and infections could become deadly.

However, it can become problematic if the inflammatory process goes on for too long or if the inflammatory response happens in areas where it is not needed. Chronic inflammation has been associated with certain illnesses such as heart disease or stroke and can lead to autoimmune disorders like rheumatoid arthritis and lupus, too. But a healthy diet and lifestyle can help to keep inflammation in control.

Heart disease and cancer were both related to inflammatory conditions. It may cause coronary blockage and a heart attack in relation to heart disease. For years, we have been told to keep our cholesterol down to prevent plaque buildup in our arteries, but scientists now agree that inflammation can play a role just as significant as cholesterol and plaque.

Inflammation is also a villain regarding cancer, especially when it comes to cancer initiation. Things are not as simple here, and inflammation definitely does not cause all cancers. Nevertheless, some of the inflammatory cells and chemicals have been shown to create mutations in DNA that can eventually lead to cancer; moreover, pre-cancer cells can also become active cancer cells. Some of the cancers considered to have been associated with inflammation are the cancer of the colon, lung, stomach, esophagus, and breast.

Inflammation also interacts with many other diseases. Both disorders of the inflammation include rheumatoid arthritis, osteoporosis, MS, lupus, emphysema, and gingivitis. Yes, any illness with a name that ends with "it is" is an inflammatory disease. Bursitis, tendonitis, arthritis, hepatitis, colitis, tonsillitis, and dermatitis are just some examples.

How inflammation Starts and progresses.

Inflammation is the corporal response to harmful stimuli. A number of things that could trigger this are:

- Pathogen infection (bacteria, viruses, etc.)

- Unintended physical injury
- Foreign objects entering the body, such as splinters, dirt or other particles
- Chemical irritants
- Frostbite and Burns
- Stress
- Toxins from air or water

In one way or another, each has experienced inflammation. The main symptoms here are redness, heat, swelling, and pain. However, in most cases, what we encounter is acute inflammation. It is a short-term process that lasts only a few days to a few weeks, and when the stimuli are removed, it mostly ceases. So, it is not critical for most people.

In contrast, chronic inflammation is inflammation that does not correctly clear up. It lasts for months, and years, even. And it can cause significant damage to your body.

However, we'll start with an overview of the acute inflammation. It goes through two main phases: a phase vascular and a phase cellular. And it consists of a series of biochemical events involving the local vascular system, the immune system, and cells within the tissue that has been injured. A brief (and simplified) outline of how this happens is:

- The process begins with the detection of some sort of harmful stimuli.

- The initial response (vascular phase) originates from cells of the immune system present in the tissue affected. One of the biggest ones which first detects it and reacts is called macrophages. They have receptors recognizing pathogens and other foreign objects (not body belongings).

- These (and other particles) macrophages release inflammation mediators that call up in other particles. Also, they release mediator molecules, including histamine, that dilate nearby blood vessels. It improves blood circulation to the area affected; the permeability (leakage) of these vessels also increases.

- The increased blood flow allows more immune cells to reach the area to fight infection. It also increases the area's amount of glucose (sugar) and oxygen to aid in nourishing the cells. At the same time, the increased vessel permeability helps bring plasma protein and antibodies-containing fluids, and so on, to the area.

- The affected area swells and turns red owing to the above. There's heating, as well, and there may be a pain.

- The cell phase begins with the increased size of the blood vessels helping white blood cells, mainly neutrophils and macrophages, migrate into the area. Once pathogens are present, they are particularly important in that they eat them, but they also play other vital roles, such as assisting in wound repair.

- One of the main things that the above buildup does is to "wall the area off" from further attack, particularly from bacteria and viruses.

- When a cleanup of dead cells and other debris begins, the pathogen (or whatever) is overcome. The start of a cycle in which new, healthy cells begin to replace the old ones, and soon the macrophages and other immune cells leave the region. And in the acute case, it all gets back to normal soon.

Cardinal Inflammatory Symptoms.

Often doctors and researchers refer by their Latin names to the five cardinal signs of inflammation:

- Dolor (pain).
- Calor (heat).
- Rubor (redness).
- Tumor (swelling).
- Functio laesa (loss of function).

Pain.

Inflammation can cause muscle and joint pain. When inflammation is chronic, a person may experience high levels of pain sensitivity and stiffness. The inflamed areas can be sensitive to contact.

Pain is the product of inflammatory chemicals that activate nerve endings, causing damage to the affected areas, with both acute and chronic inflammations.

Heat.

If inflamed areas of the body feel warm, it's because those areas have more blood flow. People with conditions of arthritis may have inflamed joints which feel warm to the touch. However, the skin around those joints may not be equally warm. Whole-body inflammation can cause fevers when someone has an illness or an infection as a result of the inflammatory response.

Redness.

Inflamed body areas can appear red in color. This is because inflamed-area blood vessels are filled with more blood than usual.

Swelling.

Swelling is common when it inflames a part of the body. It is the result of fluid accumulating throughout the body, or in the specific area affected, in tissues. Swelling can happen without inflammation, especially in the case of injuries.

Function-Loss.

Inflammation can result in loss of function, both related to injury and illness. For example, an inflamed joint can not be adequately moved, or a respiratory infection can make it difficult to breathe.

Additional Complications and Signs.

This can cause additional signs and symptoms when the inflammation is severe. This may involve a general sensation of sickness and exhaustion.

What Happens When You Experience An Inflammation?

When an inflammation occurs in your body, it can involve many different cells of the immune system. They release different substances, which are known as inflammatory mediators. These include bradykinin hormones and histamine. They cause the small blood vessels within the tissue to widen (dilate), allowing more blood to reach the tissue that has been injured. Inflamed areas turn red, and feel hot, for this reason.

The increased blood flow also allows the movement of more cells in the immune system to the damaged tissue, where they assist with the healing process. What is more, both of these hormones irritate the nerves and cause the brain to receive pain signals. This has a defensive function: If the inflammation hurts, you tend to protect the suffering part of the body.

Another function of the inflammatory mediators is to make it easier for the cells of the immune system to pass out of the small blood vessels so that more of them can enter the tissue affected. The cells of the immune system also cause more fluid to enter the inflamed tissue, which is why it frequently swells.

After a while, the swelling goes down again, when this fluid is transported out of the tissue.

Mucous membranes also release more fluid upon inflammation. This happens when you have a stuffy nose and your nose is inflamed by the membranes lining your nose. The extra fluid may then help to flush the viruses out of your body quickly.

Acute Inflammation.

Acute inflammation accompanies the knee, a sore throat, or a sprained ankle. It's a short-term solution with localized consequences, which means it operates at the exact location where a problem arises. The telltale signs of acute inflammation include swelling, redness, heat, and at times pain and loss of control, according to the National Library of Medicine (NLM).

Blood vessels dilate in the case of acute inflammation, blood flow increases, and white blood cells swarm over the injured area to facilitate healing, Dr. Scott Walker, a family practice physician at Gunnison Valley Hospital in Utah, said. This response is what turns the injured area red and gets swollen.

During the course of acute inflammation, the damaged tissue releases chemicals known as cytokines. The cytokines serve as "emergency signals" that bring immune cells, hormones, and nutrients into your body to fix the issue, Walker said.

Therefore, hormone-like substances called prostaglandins build blood clots to repair damaged tissue and, as part of the healing process, trigger pain and fever too. As the body heals, the acute inflammation slowly subsides.

Chronic Inflammation.

Chronic inflammation can have long-term and whole-body consequences as opposed to acute inflammation. Chronic inflammation is also referred to as persistent low-grade inflammation because it produces a steady, low-grade inflammation throughout the whole body, as judged by a small increase in blood or tissue-related markers of the immune system. According to a report in the Johns Hopkins Health Review, this type of systemic inflammation can contribute to disease development.

A perceived internal threat can cause low levels of inflammation, even if there is no fighting disease or healing injury, and this sometimes signals the response of the immune system. White blood cells swarm as a result but have nothing to do and can go nowhere, and eventually start attacking internal organs or other healthy tissues and cells, Walker said.

Researchers are still working on understanding the implications of chronic inflammation on the body and the mechanisms involved in the process, but many diseases are known to play a role.

For example, heart disease and stroke have been linked to chronic inflammation. One study suggests that when inflammatory cells stay in blood vessels for too long, they promote plaque buildup. The American Heart Association (AHA) states that the body perceives this plaque as a foreign material not belonging to it, so it seeks to wall off the plaque from the blood flowing within the arteries. If the plaque becomes unstable and ruptures, a clot is formed that blocks blood flow to the heart or brain and triggers a heart attack or stroke.

Another illness linked to chronic inflammation is cancer. According to the National Cancer Institute, chronic inflammation can cause damage to the DNA over time and lead to some forms of cancer.

Chronic, low-grade inflammation often has no symptoms, but doctors may test for C-reactive protein (CRP), which is a marker for blood inflammation. High CRP levels were linked to an increased risk of heart disease. According to the Mayo Clinic, CRP levels may also suggest an infection or a chronic inflammatory condition such as rheumatoid arthritis or lupus.

In addition to seeking clues in the blood, a person's diet, lifestyle habits, and exposures to the environment can contribute to chronic inflammation. In order to keep inflammation in check, it is essential to maintain a healthy lifestyle.

Chronic Inflammatory Symptoms.

One of our main goals of modern medicine is to help people avoid chronic disease and reverse it, pay a lot of attention to chronic inflammation.

Five common indications here are that somebody might have a chronic inflammatory condition.

Excessive mucus production.

Need to clear your throat or blow your nose? It sounds like you could get inflamed! In an effort to protect the epithelial cells in the respiratory system, which lead to coughing, sneezing, and a runny nose, mucous membranes contain thick phlegm when inflamed.

Rashes on the skin.

Skin rashes, like eczema or psoriasis, are inflammatory skin conditions marked by dark, rough, and flaccid skin. Both eczema and psoriasis are associated with the immune system's hypersensitivity, and individuals with these conditions are more likely to have more inflammatory mast cells that cause skin rashes to surface when triggered.

Bad digestive tract.

Common digestive problems, including bloating, abdominal pain, constipation, and loose stool may also indicate an inflammatory issue. Chronic inflammation can lead to leaky gut syndrome or intestinal permeability throughout the body, which can allow bacteria and toxins to "leak" into the rest of the body through the intestinal wall. A "leaky intestine" can intensify systemic inflammation further and lead to digestive symptoms such as abdominal distention and frequent bowel movements.

Low energy.

Feeling constantly tired despite getting enough nightly sleep is yet another sign, the body is fighting off chronic inflammation. Just as you feel run-down when you're sick, your immune system remains active when you're chronically inflamed, and works overtime to control your reaction. Its effect, chronic inflammation, raises the cellular energy demand to ensure rapid immune cell regeneration and further depletes you from the power you need to feel fully energized.

Pain in the body.

Increased systemic inflammation is commonly responsible for body pain, such as muscle aches and joint pain. When inflammatory cytokines rise in the body, muscle and joint problems can be attacked, resulting in redness, swelling, and pain. Face rashes like eczema or psoriasis

Who Is At Greatest Risk.

Firstly, it's important to point out that everyone needs to worry about out-of-control inflammation, and everyone should do what they can to improve their immune system. However, some things make some people more vulnerable to chronic inflammation and other issues with inflammation. Such are:

- Anyone who is overweight (in particular, obese). The immune system also mistakes and targets fat deposits for intruders. In fact, fat cells may leak or split open; if this occurs, macrophages come in to clean up the debris, and they may release problems-causing chemicals.

- Anybody with diabetes. Studies show that inflammation may be associated with diabetes II and that people with high rates of inflammation typically develop diabetes within a few years.

- Anybody in the family with heart disease or heart disease signs. The relationship between heart disease and chronic inflammation is complicated. It is also well known that the plaque in arteries that is the product of inflammation causes heart attacks.

- Anyone who appears to feel tired and fatigued. This is especially important when no explanation for the problem can be found. Fatigue is related to inflammation.

- Anyone who works in a toxic environment. Toxins are well known to cause unnecessary inflammation.

- Anyone that suffers from depression or anxiety greatly. Stress causes inflammation, is well known.

- Older People. When we grow older, our body changes, and we tend to produce more chemicals for inflammation and fewer chemicals for anti-inflammation.

What Can You Do To Avoid Having Chronic Inflammation.

The list below will give you a good idea of what to do to prevent chronic inflammation. However, I will list some of the important things and address them briefly. However, I should add that genes play a role in whether or not you are going to get chronic inflammation, and there is little we can do about it.

Below is a list of the major things:

- Eat a nutritious diet. It should contain at least five servings of fruits and vegetables each day. Particularly noteworthy are cruciferous vegetables; they include broccoli, cauliflower, and cabbage. Many excellent vegetables include onions, tomatoes, spinach, and beans. Some of the best fruits are citrus fruits; beers like blueberries and strawberries are essential as well. Other especially good foods are grains such as oats and whole wheat, nuts, and seeds. Even fish is essential as an omega-3 source, and you should eat it 2 to 3 times a week. You should, at the same time, avoid simple carbohydrates, fast foods, soda, saturated fats, and trans fat items.

  Don't over-consume. Often, loose weight if you're overweight.
- Get enough time. 7 hours to 8 hours is enough for most adults.
- Work out daily. In reality, exercise is a healthy way of reducing inflammation. It is important both for aerobics and weights.
- Regulate blood pressure, cholesterol, and triglycerides.
- Avoid stress.
- Avoid toxins.

The Growing Causes of Inflammation and Gut Health Relationship.

Nowadays, we hear a lot about inflammation.

In a clinical setting, we have been talking to our physicians for years about inflammation. Inflammation is the very root of the causes of chronic disease and disability, in addition to inflammation, stress, and deficiency.

It's an exciting period as a rising number of independent wellness seekers search out the root causes of their afflictions.

By the way, when we are talking about inflammation, we are talking about systemic inflammation-cellular inflammation of the body. It's not the same as twisting the knee and seeing the resulting localized swelling.

The inflammation of which we are thinking here is far more subtle. It is like a constant irritant to our minds and bodies... Like a fire burning silently inside.

Tackling intestinal inflammation is of particular importance. As cutting-edge scientific research continues to demonstrate, the gut is intricately related to brain and brain function. A "bad intestine is equivalent to a bad brain" Consider the potential to treat (or prevent) problems such as depression, anxiety, spectrum disorders, Alzheimer's, and so forth more effectively and successfully. No need to forget the heart.

So, what causes inflammation?

Here are some of the most important inflammatory factors:

- Drug Use- Many over-the-counter and prescription drugs directly contribute to the inflammation itself. NSAIDS (non-steroidal anti-inflammatory medications like Aspirin, Ibuprofen, Celebrex, etc.) is one of these. Research clearly shows that even taking over-the-counter drugs like ibuprofen for three days can cause inflammation and leaky intestines. Another family medication that is directly associated with inflammation of the gut is antibiotics. Not only do antibiotics kill the intended target bacteria-they wreak havoc on all bacteria, including the "clean" bacteria that are so important to our overall health and immune function in our intestinal systems.

- Nutritional deficiencies — As I mentioned earlier, deficiency means that we don't get what our cells need to achieve and/or sustain a homeostatic cell function state. This can lead to inflammation due to the absence of the main' ingredients' needed for proper digestion.

- Leaky Gut and Autoimmune Disorders - I know I just listed this, but this list deserves its own distinct location. It is a vicious cycle: leaky intestines contribute to inflammation... That results in leaky gut... That results in increased inflammation. You get that impression. In fact, this is an immune response. The immune system actually does its job by removing objects that are not supposed to be there, such as excessively large molecules that move through the intestinal barrier. The stage is set beautifully for an autoimmune condition as the immune response proceeds on its battle "against" the body as this cycle continues. The smart approach to fixing this is NOT to inhibit the overall immune response, but to (1) eliminate the causes, 'calm' the immune response, and (2) repair the intestine.

- Stress-Chronic - stress plays a direct role in cellular inflammation, whether it is mental, emotional, or physical. Our bodies are ideally suited for short stress bursts -it's called the "fight or flight response." But, when we're subjected to chronic stress, processes break down. This can be due to ongoing financial issues, relationship difficulties, job frustration, chronic lack of sleep, injury, overwork, over-training (for example, for a marathon), medications, toxic foods... Stressors aren't missing! Stress creates a unique sequence of neuro-hormonal activities that can not easily be ignored within the brain and body.

- Toxicity-Toxicity overflows us. We should respond to some of that. We can not do some of that. Toxicity causes a distinct chemical / hormonal reaction in the brain and sets off a chain of events all over the body... One such inflammation. Look at the list in the category "pain"- these are all toxicity sources. We may add environmental toxicity to that list too. Find air, water, personal care products, kitchen, greenhouse, and lawn care products, cosmetics, heavy metals, vaccines, etc. sources of toxicity. Considering just how unhealthy our culture has become, maybe daunting. (That's why I think a regular cell detoxification protocol is so important). Diet-Eating foods that are "inflammatory," especially grains such as wheat, barley, and rye that contain gluten and introduce inflammatory proteins called prolamins. Such irritate the stomach regularly and lead to the permeability of the gut or "leaky intestine." Once the intestine is too permeable, it allows large molecules that were never meant to move through the intestinal barrier. This activates an over-active immune response as the immune system is, so to speak, heading into the attack. Inflammation is one consequence of this heightened immune reaction.

- Sugar-Whether it's the white powdery, crystal stuff right off the spoon or straight out of a bottle, or foods and drinks that break down to sugar quickly in our bloodstream (such as soda, candy, sweets and starchy carbs such as bread, pasta, cereal, crackers, pizza, baked goods, and pastries) sugar spikes create an overall negative response. Dysregulation of the blood sugar from persistent spikes in sugar and insulin resistance are major contributors to inflammation. Clearly, artificial sweeteners are no option! These are extremely toxic and also lead to inflammation.

- Chronic alcohol consumption-Alcohol leads to leaky gut as well as to overgrowth of bacteria and fungal / yeast in the intestines. It is also a highly concentrated dose of sugar, which activates the response of the body to insulin.

- Low Stomach Hydrochloric Acid-Most people think indigestion and acid reflux are the results of having too much stomach acid. Actually, it's just the opposite, most of the time, particularly as we get older. When we don't have enough HCL to break down our food properly, we will feel the burning sensation when food particles that aren't properly broken down remain in the upper digestive tract for longer than they should (because the body says "oh, this food is too large for me to move along to the small intestines!"). And, if these excessively large food particles are passed on to the small intestine, they cause the intestinal lining to break down, leading to the leaky intestine, causing chronic inflammation.

(So, those acid pumps that inhibit drugs you see on TV? They end up causing the food to be forced out of the stomach before it breaks down efficiently-so you stop feeling burning-but now you've set the stage for much bigger problems with intestinal permeability, leaky gut, inflammation, and setting the stage for the autoimmune disease over time.) 12. Hormonal Imbalance-This one is big! We're not just thinking about reproductive hormones, or the "women's" hormones that many people often believe when you mention the word "hormonal!" Hormones are the chemical messengers for all of our bodies ' processes, and they play a critical role in all functions. One example of the link between hormonal-inflammation is cortisol, the stress hormone.

When chronic stress or toxicity tires our adrenal system, we can burn through so much of our supply of the stress hormone that cortisol is depleted. Unfortunately, cortisol is one of the things our body, naturally, uses to regulate the inflammatory process!

On the flip side, the hormonal receptors on the cell membrane do not end up being so' receptive' to the hormonal message attempting to be transmitted when there is inflammation. This obviously contributes to a hormonal dysregulation-the message can not reach its intended destination, or the message gets distorted. A medicine or cream containing hormones doesn't fix this problem.

- "Bad" Fats-Another guilty dietary. These are trans fats, hydrogenated and partially hydrogenated fats, consumer vegetable oils, polluted animal fat, and so on. These help an inflammatory state. Stick to pure coconut oil, natural grass-fed butter, organic extra virgin olive oil, balanced grass-fed, and free-range animal fats, wild fish, healthy fat foods such as avocado, omega-3 to omega-6 fat balance, and so on. Usually, the "bad" fats are what we get from junk food, fast food, restaurant food, fried food, and so on. Even when we start with "good" food, the results are toxic and inflammatory when cooked with bad fats.

- Deprivation of Chronic Sleep-Hopefully, you can see the connection here... Deprivation (or deficiency) anywhere along with the' things our body needs' continuum will result in a toxic, inflamed situation. But even one night of sleep deprivation (we're talking about 4-5 hours of sleep here) has been shown to increase the inflammation markers dramatically!

- Infections-Bacterial, bacterial, parasitic, or fungal. Such chronic infections, often undetected and untreated, cause inflammation as the immune system is on the offensive without relent, trying to keep the infection under control. One of the simplest things we can do to offset potential infection, particularly in the gut, is to replenish the gut in the form of high-quality probiotics with healthy, immune-enhancing bacteria.

- Severe Brain Trauma-Remember the vital link between the intestine and the brain? Here, the opposite plays out. When a brain injury occurs, that, in turn, has been shown to cause leaky intestine in as little as six hours or less! It, of course, leads to chronic inflammation over time unless handled appropriately.

How Is One Diagnosed With Inflammation?

There is no single test diagnosis of inflammation or triggering conditions. Instead, your doctor can give you any of the tests below to make a diagnosis based on your symptoms.

Blood tests Some so-called markers help to detect inflammation in the body. Certain markers are non-specific, however, which means that abnormal rates will indicate that something is wrong, but not what is wrong.

Serum protein electrophoresis (SPE).

SPE is regarded as the best way to confirm chronic inflammation using Reliable Source. To detect any issues, it tests those proteins in the liquid portion of the blood. Too much or too little of those proteins may contribute to inflammation and markers for other conditions.

Erythrocyte sedimentation rate (ESR).

Occasionally, the ESR test is considered a measure of sedimentation rate. This test measures inflammation indirectly by calculating the rate at which the red blood cells sink in a blood tube. The quicker they sink, the more likely you get inflamed.

The ESR test is rarely performed alone, as it does not help to identify unique inflammatory causes. Instead, it can help the doctor determine that there is inflammation. It can allow them to track your condition too.

C-reactive protein (CRP).

In response to inflammation, CRP is naturally produced in the liver. Because of several inflammatory conditions, a high level of CRP can occur in your blood.

Although this test is highly sensitive to inflammation, it does not help to differentiate between acute and chronic inflammation, as CRP will be elevated during both. High levels combined with some symptoms can help make a diagnosis for your doctor.

Plasma viscosity.

The test measures blood thickness. Inflammation or infection may make plasma thicken.

Other blood tests.

If your doctor believes that the inflammation is due to viruses or bacteria, they may do more specific tests. In this situation, your doctor will speak with you about what to expect.

Other diagnostic tests.

If you have some symptoms, such as chronic diarrhea or numbness on one side of your face, your doctor might ask for an imaging test to check certain parts of your body or brain. Widespread use is of MRIs and X-rays.

Your doctor may perform a procedure to look inside parts of the digestive tract to diagnose inflammatory gastrointestinal conditions. Those tests might include:

Sigmoidoscopy, colonoscopy, upper endoscopy.

Anti-Aging And Inflammation.

Inflammation is mainly a well-functioning immune system that activates a complex series of chemical and cellular activities performed by the body in response to (1) damage or (2) physical, chemical, or biological stimulation. We've both heard of inflammation, felt its painful, and treated it in our usual ways. But many of us don't know there is a direct connection between inflammation and aging. They are not aware that free radicals within our bodies are responsible for inflammation and the factors that cause these free radicals in our daily lives that can disrupt cell function. This segment will help explain that the secret cause of aging and disease is the constant inflammation endured during your lifetime. It will investigate the causes of inflammation and will provide ways to manage these irregular cellular activities through diet and supplementation, maintaining a healthy lifestyle for managing age.

Aging is inevitable, but a choice is how one ages. Some people seem to age well, they look younger than their actual date of birth; others seem a decade older than their chronological age. Our genetic makeup helps to decide how we age, but other factors are equally important. Medical intervention has been instrumental in extending lifespan. Although the average lifespan in 1900 was around 46 to 48 years, today, people can expect to live well into their 80s. But how one lives these years and how well one keeps chronic disease at bay, heavily depends on anti-aging factors.

The "free radical aging theory" explores the factors that affect our genes and provides a basis for how we age. The theory explains in simple terms how mutations occur and how we can avoid and solve aging problems resulting from injury, illness, or DNA damage. The message is that free radicals are the main cause of inflammation within the body, contributing to illness. Control free radical damage through dietary choices and antioxidant supplementation, and you control DNA damage.

Denham Harman, a pioneer in medical physics at the University of California, Berkeley, developed in 1956 the "free radical theory of aging" Free radicals are heavily charged atoms which lack one electron, rendering them unstable. We come into our body through sunlight, poor diet, drug use, tobacco use, airborne chemicals, even stressing, and stealing an electron to achieve chemical stability. The favored targets are fatty acids, phospholipid-rich cell membranes, DNA, and proteins. When targeted cellular orderly processes are replaced by the utter chaos of electron swapping, which eventually disrupts the function of the cell. Free radicals are known to be the primary culprits in aging because they induce spontaneous radical change and deviation from a well-ordered natural cellular metabolism. As a consequence, free radicals create inflammation, and the cause of aging and disease is regular inflammation maintained over a lifetime. Other inflammatory symptoms include swelling, heat, joint pain, and redness. When we age, our defenses weaken, and the end products of oxidative damage accumulate in our tissues. We note that our skin is cracking, or maybe we are developing "age spots." Oxidative stress on the inside of our body destroys main molecules important to our DNA, causing cancer, diabetes, heart disease, poor circulation, and other age-related diseases.

DNA is especially prone to oxidative stress. They leave "pits" in the individual DNA strands, as electrons are stolen. Free radicals create a split and wear off of DNA strands. The resulting nicks and strand breaks affect the working cells as well as the stem cells. Damage to stem cells is extremely devastating, as these cells are precursors to thousands of different types of cells found within the body. Since reproduction is the primary role of stem cells, the damaged stem cells affect all working cells in future generations. Cancer is one condition which depends on the damage to DNA. The many types of skin cancer are a common example of this.

Inflammation is an essential mechanism of protection of the body's immune system. Once a foreign body is identified, the immune system reacts with inflammation at the site of the infection, marked by redness, swelling, and pain. Inflammation causes the same things which activate free radicals. The causes of inflammation include radiation, smog, airborne pollutants, poor diet, alcohol, medications, smoking, and stress. Acute inflammation develops after an injury or infection. This step usually resolves itself within a 24 to 48 hour period, and the recovery process begins. Cellular debris is eliminated from the injury site and the development of healthy replacement tissue. Our antioxidant defenses weaken as we age, and the oxidant damage triggers chronic inflammatory conditions. This form of inflammation is extended further. Free radicals, severe stress, and agents for the atmosphere do not respond to immune attacks. There is no recovery process, and there is severe damage to the pain and tissue. Efficient DNA repair depends on overcoming these conditions and reversing aging. Our question is, how can we support nature through a cycle of DNA repair and reverse aging? One way is by taking diet and supplementing. Another way of doing that is how you live your life. All methods reflect choices.

Appropriate choices in diet, nutrition, and lifestyle are necessary to prevent inflammation, to neutralize free radicals, and to promote healthy age management. Acid and alkaline based foods are among our options. Diet would consist of 80%

alkaline foods and 20% acidic foods. A rainbow variety of six fruit and vegetable portions, organic wherever possible, will ensure this all essential acid / alkaline balance reduces inflammation by supplying a multitude of antioxidants for the body. Carrots, onions, mangos, pumpkin, peppers, and papaya are all orange and' red-coded' and protect our DNA. Asparagus, broccoli, bok choy, onions, and mustard greens are 'color-coded' and contribute to enhancing cellular nutrition and detoxifying our body. Blackberries, beets, cherries, are purple and blue, and the inflammation is that. Barley, mushrooms, tofu, and wild rice are tan and reduce insulin resistance and hormone balance. To neutralize free radicals, herbs, and spices such as garlic, turmeric, cinnamon, curry, ginger, and cayenne aid.

Meats, plants, nuts, and sugar are usually acidic and foster toxic, free radicals. Meats should be free-range, so they are hormone-free and antibiotic-free. One should have a salmon, tilapia, flounder, and sardines raised farm diet and avoid swordfish that is considered to be high in mercury. Barley, quinoa, brown rice, and wild rice represent excellent grain options. Nuts and seeds are important to a well-rounded diet. With each meal, dark leafy greens, legumes, and red, yellow, orange, and green vegetables must be eaten in order to balance the essential acidic foods that provide us with the much-needed protein vitamins and minerals our body needs.

Through high levels of alkaline water intake, green tea, and avoiding sugar, vinegar, salt, and corn syrup, we can further reduce inflammation. In a nutshell, prioritize lean organic protein, mix vegetable sources, eat selectively, avoid sugar candy, nitrates, nitrites, smoked meats, and trans-fats, track portion sizes, not eat on the road, and chew your food. You should have five fruit and vegetable portions; ideally, a combination of green and orange-red colors. Drink plenty of water between meals; do not consume soda, eat meals regularly; do not eat late, and stop food processing. Reduce dairy intake. We are the only organisms eating any other kind of milk!

Many anti-inflammatory supplements are antioxidants which help our body control radical damage free of charge. Multivitamin/mineral complex of high quality is essential for a healthy lifestyle. Folic acids, B vitamins, vitamins D, C, A, E, Boswella, Glucosamine-Chondroitin, Curcumin, molecularly purified Omega 3 and 6 from cold-water fish Tri-Methylglycine, CoQ Enzyme 10, R-Lipoic Acid, and Resveratrol, are all supplements that will slow the development of the disease and reduce inflammation. Vitamins A, C, and E reduce the risk of developing heart disease. They reduce inflammation and defend against oxidative damage arising from it. Those with diabetes can see "insulin function," improving Green tea protects against estrogenic breast cancer. Vitamin D3 prevents colon cancer, and aged garlic prevents DNA damage, and reduces inflammation as well. In general, we rid our bodies of free radicals through detoxification.

The use of the CoQ10 enzyme has important outcomes in curbing aging. This drug prevents oxidative brain damage, improves accelerated heart attack recovery and heart function, and prevents thyroid disorders. Alpha-Lipoic acid enhances the metabolism of carbohydrates, improves brain energy and muscle-skeletal strength, and soaks up free radicals within the body.

Diet, nutrition, and education are the most important ingredients in age management. Yet changes in lifestyle complete the whole picture of encouraging lifespan. Research shows that stress triggers profound changes in cellular structure, leading to aging diseases, especially those involving inflammation and immune function. Act to alleviate depression and extend your lifespan. Daily exercise, prayer, and meditation are also constructive influences that can be incorporated into one's life. Learn to be wise, develop a relationship with your God and think "holistically" Reduce alcohol consumption, assist with probiotics in your digestive process, establish proper disposal, and reduce acidic foods. There is no magic bullet, but a desire for health becomes a lifestyle that provides essential gifts for a life of good feeling and good looking—real beauty springs from within. There is no shortcut!

The Immune System, Cancer, And Inflammation.

The immune system is a beautiful cell system and signals cytokines which battle infections and keep us healthy. Every day we come into contact with milliards of microorganisms. These include parasites, bacteria, viruses, and fungi. We have an immune system to protect us. The immune system is a complex array of pathogens that combats white blood cells and the complement system and cytokines from their partners.

The supplement system includes small proteins that circulate all over the blood system. Their role is to identify and bind foreign substances (antigens) and then activate the rest of the system. They stick with and label the bad cells so that the other immune cells can identify the infectious cells. Killing bacteria is another function of the complement system.

The next community is that of phagocytes. Some cells that eat a process called phagocytosis of bacteria. The phagocytes include granulocytes, transformed monocyte macrophages, and dendritic cells. This cell layer provides the first line of defense against infections.

The next collection includes lymphocytes. There are numerous lymphocyte types, and each has a specific function. T-helper cells are relevant immune system regulators. When they get in touch with a cell presenting an antigen like a macrophage that has just eaten a bacteria, the helper cell is activated, and then it helps to turn the rest of the immune system on. Another T-cell type is that of a T-cell killer. Such cells circulate in the body finding pathogens or healthy infected cells or even cancer cells. Their job is pretty easy; they kill him when they find a bad cell. Through producing immunoglobulins, B-lymphocytes help the immune system destroy bacteria. Immunoglobulins serve as tags labeling the phagocytes for the removal of bacteria. These are created whenever you get an infection or a vaccine. The B-lymphocytes recall when the same bug invades the body, and then develop more immunoglobulins through the plasma cells to help kill the virus.

Substances are called cytokines, at last. These substances are used for a range of uses. They help each other signal the cells; they can act as growth factors, they recruit immune cells, they activate immune cells, they shut off immune cells, and some even act as hormones. To keep the system running, the cytokines are very critical, and they need to be in balance. Some cytokines switch the system on and turn off. When an imbalance exists, either an immune deficiency or an overactive immune system is the result. The overactive immune system is what chronic inflammation means, and this is a bad thing because of the causes of chronic inflammation diseases. Chronic inflammation has previously been involved in heart disease, stroke, diabetes, and cancer.

Cancer And Inflammation.

We have learned about inflammation and cancer since the discovery of white blood cells in tumor tissues by Rudolph Virchow in 1863. Today the connection between chronic inflammation and cancer is widely accepted. Several common examples of chronic inflammation cancers include ulcerative colitis and Crohn's disease that leads to cancer of the intestine. Barrett's esophagus results in esophageal cancer. Celiac disease can lead to lymphomas in the small intestine. Hashimoto's thyroiditis can result in thyroid lymphoma.

Inflammation induces all stages of tumor development; initiation, progression, and metastasis. The growth of tumors is the process where a normal cell becomes malignant. Tumor development is the mechanism by which the cancer cell develops, and metastasis is the process by which the cancer cell spreads through the lymph nodes to distant organs, either through the lymph nodes or through the blood.

In tumor cell initiation, the function of inflammation is clear, but the mechanism is not yet being worked out. It is known to be a two-part process. The responsibility for secreting reactive oxygen species (ROS) and reactive nitrogen species (RNS) rests with the inflammatory cells. These are usually used to destroy normal cells that are infected with bacteria or viruses. Such ROS and RNS can damage the DNA of normal cells and cause mutations in a chronic state. The initial process can be a mutation in an oncogene, which eventually leads to cancer. The second step is to secrete cytokines from the inflammatory cells that accelerate cell growth, so not only are the cells stimulated to develop, but they do so in an environment full of ROS and RNS that creates a perfect situation to generate mutated oncogenes.

The way chronic inflammation promotes the proliferation of tumor cells is not well explained. Inflammatory cytokines are thought to produce many effects, especially promoting growth and tissue degradation surrounding the tumor (stromal matrix), which helps tumor cells spread and migrate.

Finally, the cytokine milieu also promotes metastasis. Some of these function as growth factors for the development of blood vessels. This is called angiogenesis, and metastasizing is necessary for tumor cells. In addition, as the blood vessels develop around the tumor cell, additional cytokines have protease activity that breaks down the stromal matrix and help the cancer cells to move into the blood vessel and then metastasize.

When the immune system functions properly, we remain protected from diseases and cancers in the best of health. Our best defense is a balanced immune system, but what is the best food for your immune system? Here's a list, and it's safer, as always, to get those nutrients directly from food rather than a tablet.

The Best Immune-Boosting Nutrients.

- ***Vitamin C:*** Increases white blood cell production, antibodies, and interferon production; A mere 200 mg/day is needed. Big doses end up in the toilet. Taking your vitamin C from citrus fruits, green peppers, bananas, tomatoes, broccoli, and sweet and white potatoes is the best option.
- ***Vitamin E:*** increases the role of naturally occurring killer cells and B cells. It can be found in fruits, seeds, and oils.
- ***Carotenoids:*** Vitamin A and beta-carotene improve cell-fighting infections and are potent antioxidants. The anti-cancer activity has also been found and can be found in green leafy vegetables, brightly colored vegetables, shrimp, fish, eggs, and dairy products.
- ***Bioflavonoids:*** are antiviral and anti-inflammatory. They strengthen the cell walls and are essential for

vitamin C absorption. Bioflavonoids can be present on the citrus fruits alongside vitamin C.

- **Zinc:** Improves white blood cell production, particularly for T cells. Zinc has been shown to a period of the common cold in clinical studies. Zinc can be found in peanuts, peas, lentils, and lima beans.
- **Garlic:** It enhances white blood cells, natural killer cells, and antibody development. It has strong antibacterial effects, as well. Try to add garlic to your diet whenever possible.
- **Selenium:** Increases the cells that battle against natural killer cells and cancer. There is some positive proof of its ability to prevent cancer.
- **Omega-3 fatty acids:** It is an excellent fat. It is anti-inflammatory, linked to good heart health, boosts the immune system, especially the phagocytes, and has anti-cancer effects.
- **Mushrooms:** renowned in the Orient for centuries for their immune-stimulating qualities. Reishi, Maitake, and Shiitake strengthen the immune system and combat cancer-like diseases.

Inflammation, and Disease.

There is a mechanism in the body which medical experts now believe to be involved in all documented processes of disease from heart disease to cancer to Alzheimer's disease-inflammation. Some of you'll have had an infection before. Ever have you had a splinter in your finger? It became red and swollen, it may have bled a little, and it definitely was hot and uncomfortable-all the classic signs of inflammation. Today, inflammation is, in reality, a normal response to such an injury, and it serves us well. This helps kill bacteria, parasites, and viruses that try to infect us, and that inflammation keeps us alive. This form of inflammation usually shows a 100fold increase in markers of the immune system, such as white blood cells and cytokines such as IL-6, alpha TNF, or reactive protein C (CRP).

There is, however, another, more profound inflammatory response in the body-what Dr. Barry Sears calls "silent inflammation." This form of inflammation does not cause the pain, swelling, redness, and heat associated with classic inflammation. It can only display a 4-5 fold increase in markers of the immune system, so it can often be difficult to detect. Development may take years or even decades, which slowly but surely damages DNA and leads to illness. Sadly this form of silent inflammation is not treated very well by modern medicine. It is the result of poor lifestyle choices, and a much better approach to improve lifestyle and diet than to use anti-inflammatory drugs.

Multi-factorial: The causes of silent inflammation.

- Too much alcohol.
- Poor diet.
- Inactivity.
- Pollution.
- Poor sleep.
- Stress / Strain.
- Drug use.

Excess body fat is one of the primary sources of mute inflammation in the body. Fat is not only an unsightly inert material that lies on your love handles or top of your muffins. It does not just serve as a pool of energy to be invoked when energy is needed. Fat is metabolic tissue that can cause the body to have all sorts of things happen. Fat cells are infected with high levels of immune cells releasing inflammatory chemicals that interfere with sugar intake and fat burning in liver cells that lead to insulin resistance, type 2 diabetes onset, and narrowing arteries. Fat cells release chemicals that coagulate the blood, increase blood pressure, and convert inactive stress hormones into active stress hormones and lead to conditions such as hypertension, stroke, cardiovascular disease, and PCOS.

Inflammation And Cardiac Disease.

Now, for many of you, this may be a little out there, mainly as we've been brainwashed into believing that saturated fat and cholesterol blocks arteries and causes heart attacks. But what researchers are now finding out is that perhaps the major player here is inflammation, not cholesterol.

As I said, when there is harm to the body, the inflammatory response gets mobilized. Sadly from free radicals, the body is under constant low-level oxidative damage all the time. These free radicals are nasty little unstable molecules that fly around stealing electrons from the cells and causing havoc in general. The resistance of the body to these free radicals is antioxidants; antioxidants can safely donate their electrons to the free radicals to make them safe. Amino acids and nutrients such as vitamin A, vitamin C, vitamin E, calcium, selenium, and many other compounds like alpha-lipoic acid, green tea extract, and carotenes form the primary source of antioxidants in our body.

The classic definition of heart disease is somewhat like this:

- Too much cholesterol in the diet, such as coronary arteries, allows cholesterol to be stored in the arteries.

- Deposited cholesterol in the coronary arteries causes arteries to narrow or obstruct, and hey presto a heart attack.

  This looks like a novel approach to heart disease involving inflammation: a poor diet that lacks antioxidants contributes to weak defense from free radicals and oxidative damage.
- As cholesterol flows in and out of the vascular epithelial cells through the arteries, it passes.
- Free radicals invade cholesterol and "oxidized cholesterol" gets damaged
- The immune system, which conducts an inflammatory reaction by which immune cells called macrophages come along and consume the oxidized cholesterol, does not accept oxidized cholesterol.
- The macrophage that has consumed the damaged cholesterol becomes a foam cell that is now lodged within the epithelial cells, lining the artery walls.
- As these foam cells build up, they cause the artery to narrow and may result in reduced blood flow to the heart muscle.
- Yeah, a heart attack is imminent.

And cholesterol appears just to be the innocent bystander of the oxidative damage done by a diet that lacks antioxidants.

Find these few studies to stress the point:

In 2008 the JUPITER report surveyed 17,000 people who were not considered at risk for heart disease. This book examined whether the Crestor statin drug could prevent heart disease in healthy individuals with low levels of LDL cholesterol but elevated CRP (a proxy for inflammation).

The study found "unambiguous evidence of reduced cardiovascular morbidity and mortality (approximately 40 percent) among those treated with statin compared to placebo" Which process was there at work, however? We know the study group had low cholesterol, so reducing it, even more, was improving, or lowering CRP statins and avoiding heart disease by reducing inflammation.

This study called The Lyon Diet Heart Research studied 600 individuals who had survived a first heart attack and were at high risk from another. The authors separate one of two classes:

Group 1 No dietary intervention was offered.
Group 2 received advice (more on this later) to adopt a Mediterranean diet.

What were the outcomes? Well, as with the JUPITER case, The Lyon Diet Heart Study was also stopped early because those who adopted the Mediterranean diet had such a significant reduction in repeated heart attacks that the authors felt ethically compelled to place everyone on a

Mediterranean diet. Those still eating a Mediterranean diet had a 50-70% lower risk of repeated heart attacks after 4 years! Compare this to the JUPITER study in which those taking a drug had only a 40% reduction in cardiovascular morbidity, and it is quite clear that making significant changes in your diet and lifestyle are far more effective in preventing heart disease than taking medication.

The Mediterranean diet.

In general, the Mediterranean diet is considered a natural diet of Crete's inhabitants between 1945 and 1970. It is composed of the following foods:

- Plant food (fruits, vegetables, pulses, beans and lentils, whole grains, nuts, and seeds) is plentiful.
- A typical daily snack is fresh fruit.
- Olive oil is the main source of fat.
- Less than 8 percent of the total calories are saturated fat.
- Strong dairy products, primarily cheese, and yogurt.
- The fish, lamb, and poultry are moderate.
- Low red meat.
- Less than 4 eggs a week.
- 1 or 2 glasses of wine a day.
- Just under 2000 calories a day.

This diet may be moderate to low in saturated fat, but it is high in omega 3 fats, fibers, and antioxidants that help prevent inflammation.

Inflammation And High Blood Pressure.

The "silent inflammation" of Dr. Barry Sears leads not only to heart disease but also to high blood pressure or what is also called hypertension. Now, hypertension is somewhat a rare disease because, in the early stages, there are no visible signs, so it's better to check your blood pressure and do everything you can to keep it in the "natural" range.

Many of you are going to go to the GP and have your blood pressure checked. You may have been told you have a blood pressure of 120 over 80 or 135 over 90, but what does that number mean?

It drives blood out into the arteries as the heartbeats, which creates the first number in a reading of BP. That number should be 120mmHg, which is considered normal. It would be considered bad to be any higher than 140mmHg. Conversely, if that number is too small, it can be bad also. However, if the arteries were not robust or created any resistance to the blood pressure being pumped out by the heart, then the arteries would break open. This resistance that the arteries produce is the second number in a reading of BP. That number should be 80mmHg, which is considered normal. The higher the 90mmHg would be regarded as bad, the other way round if that number is too low, it can be bad as well.

They can make predictions of your life expectancy based on your blood pressure from scientific research. As you can see, the higher the blood pressure, the shorter your life expectancy is.

- 130/90 BP= 67 1/2 years.
- 140/95 bp= 62 1/2 years.
- 150/100 BP= 55 years.

The arteries are not just detailed static channels that the blood flows, and they are capable of constricting and dilating depending on various factors such as stress, smoking, and nutritional status. If a tube through which a fluid passes narrows, the pressure in that tube increases, the pressure in the tube decreases, much like what happens in the bloodstream, conversely if it widens.

Many of you will have learned that if you're overweight or consume too much salt, you'll have higher blood pressure, and you need to minimize salt in the diet to lower blood pressure- true, but this isn't the only mechanism at work here.

Inflammation plays a significant role in high blood pressure too.

We need to learn a little bit about vascular biology to understand this (I can see your eyes glazing over but bear with me). The arteries are lined with cells called endothelial cells, which produce a host of chemicals capable of constricting or dilating your arteries. One of the main vasodilators released by endothelial cells is nitric oxide, and mostly, nitric oxide allows the arteries to relax and expand, thus lowering blood pressure. What we know is that C-reactive protein (CRP) that I mentioned earlier will reduce endothelial nitric oxide production and increase inflammatory nitric oxide, leading to vasoconstriction and increased blood pressure. Nitric oxide is essentially devoured by inflammation. They also recognize that oxidative damage and free radicals suppress nitric oxide and that patients with hypertension have decreased antioxidants such as glutathione, superoxide dismutase, vitamin E, vitamin C, vitamin A, copper, and polyunsaturated fats.

So, you have it there-inflammation causes blood pressure to increase.

One item shown to lower blood pressure is something called the diet DASH (Dietary Approaches to Stop Hypertension). In fact, the DASH diet is a pinch of low salt, low carb diet that is higher in protein and essential fats.

- Meat poultry and oily fish two to four servings a day.
- 6-8 servings of vegetables per day.
- 4 Servings of fruits a day.
- Dried beans, seeds, and nuts 1-2 daily portions.
- Low-fat dairy products one or two servings a day.
- 1-2 servings of cereals, grains, and pasta a day.
- Fats and oils 4-5 servings per day (mainly unsaturated fats such as olive oil, fish oil, but some saturated fat is permissible).
- Fiber-50g per day (mix of soluble and insoluble fiber- may require a fiber supplement).

Once, this diet is lower in inflammatory foods and higher in antioxidants, much like the former Mediterranean diet (in fact, there are many similarities).

Inflammation and Cancer.

A growing number of cancer researchers conclude that cancer is essentially an inflammatory disease and that the longer a tissue or organ involves inflammation, the higher the risk of subsequent carcinogenesis.

Epidemiological studies suggest that about 15 percent of all cancers worldwide are correlated with a microbial infection, including cervical and HPV1 viruses, bowel cancer, and inflammatory bowel disease attributable to bacterial dysbiosis and secondary stomach cancer. Infection with a Pylori. All of these infectious agents require an inflammatory response in the body.

One way the immune system deals with these threats is to unleash free radicals that kill the bacteria and invading viruses. Such free radicals, however, can also damage healthy cell DNA. Those cells either heal or die. If a large number of cells in an area die due to infection, an inflammatory mediated response may result in the growth of the tumor.

Many other cancers, such as smoking and lung cancer or chemical toxicity (xenoestrogens) and breast cancer, can result from long-term chronic discomfort and inflammation. DNA injury, inflammatory cell death, and tumor growth are again present.

Ultimately these tumors are able to release inflammatory substances that can sustain their growth, such as by promoting the development of new blood vessels to support tumor growth.

I will not be discussing an "anti-cancer" diet, but I will suggest that sugar can be a contributing cause to cancer. Cancer likes sugar, which seems to be being banded around. Cancer cells tend to use a mixture of lots of sugar and different proteins to ignore cellular instructions for dying off and continuing to grow. We also know that people who eat more omega-3 fats, antioxidants, and fiber are less affected by cancer. So eating an anti-inflammatory diet will protect you from cancer by eating such a diet rich in oily fish, fruits, and vegetables.

Inflammation and Diabetes.

Even inflammation could be a cause of type 2 diabetes. This form of diabetes is generally regarded as the result of being overweight and consuming too much sugar, which makes the cells resistant to insulin effects.

But what the cause could actually be, is... inflammation!

I have already addressed how overweight causes a lot of inflammatory chemicals to be released that lead to what Dr. Barry Sears terms "silent inflammation." Well, mice research shows that inflammation caused by immune cells called macrophages (the same cells that become foam cells that contribute to blocked arteries-and concentrated in fat cells as well) contributes to insulin resistance and type 2 diabetes.

This research was done in genetically engineered mice that lacked a specific gene present in the pancreatic insulin-producing cells. These genes are immune to the inflammatory response caused by macrophages, and they did not develop diabetes when these mice lacked the gene, even when fed an extremely high-fat diet.

Now this research has been done in mice, and it needs to be taken cautiously to apply it to humans. However, there is a good argument for reducing inflammation to protect the pancreas.

Other anti-inflammatory foods which can help to protect yourself from "silent inflammation" include:

- Oily fish, which is high in omega 3 fats.
- Ginger.
- Garlic.
- Turmeric.
- Quercitin occurs in ointments, broccoli, tea, wine, and raisins.

Foods That Promote Inflammation.

"The more severe the pain or disease, the more serious the necessary changes will be, which may involve breaking bad habits, or developing new and better ones." -Peter McWilliams. You are not powerless in your battle against inflammation! The diet plays a major role in activating or suppressing the inflammatory-causing protein called cytokines.

The following are food groups you can avoid because they send out a signal to your body to create more inflammatory cytokines. These are also harmful to your body in many ways, polluting the body's inner environment and inducing inflammation.

Most Meat, Except Oily Fish.

The expression "all things in moderation" is often used. Meat is an exception to this rule, especially red meat. Also, what most would find a "normal" amount of red meat could produce an excessive number of cytokines and cause symptoms of autoimmune disease.

The "low-carb craze" has caused an increase in meat consumption for some. When consuming the low-carb way means you're eating a lot of foods, the autoimmune condition is getting worse. Meat protein raises blood levels of the uric acid and urea toxins. To help flush out those toxins, the body pumps large amounts of water into the kidneys. Swift-water "weight loss" is the product of a high animal-based protein diet. The cons of this "weight loss" is that it causes loss of essential minerals to the body. Mineral imperfections cause autoimmunity. A better choice of protein comes from proteins dependent on the vegetables. Such proteins enhance the preservation of minerals within the body.

One doctor has confirmed that most of his lupus patients did not eat meat within two weeks, showing significant improvement in their skin lesions.

The Swank Diet calls for a year of giving up red meat, then giving yourself four ounces of red meat per week after the first year. This diet has significantly improved the lives of people with Multiple Sclerosis (MS). For thirty years, Dr. Swank observed over 150 of his MS patients. Those who followed the diet died at a rate of 5%, while patients who did not follow his diet had a death rate of about 85% over the same period.

Reducing meat intake, though, is not only about living longer, it is about living well! This advice is for everybody, not just those whose set of autoimmune symptoms is called lupus or

MS. Eating red meat will raise their numbers no matter where the cytokines accumulate in your body or what they strike. It also makes a difference in the way the meat is cooked. Charbed and grilled meats of any kind are far worse for you and should be avoided absolutely.

Fish is the food rule exception. Fish do not elevate cytokine levels. Indeed it eliminates them. The concern is that radioactive mercury contaminates a large part of our fish. Unless you're confident that your food supply is mercury-free, you can limit your intake of fish to one serving per week instead of using fish oil supplements. Some may even become prone to one infected fish serving. Check your local health food groceries for fish farmed in water certified as "mercury-free." Furthermore, salmon is a readily available food that is least likely to be polluted with mercury.

Egg Yolks.

Egg yolks are rich in arachidonic acid, and dairy products. This is the same material that inflammates meats so much. If you are eating eggs, you can eat only the whites. Eggs can be identified on a food label as albumin, globulin, ovomucin, or as vitellin.

Dairy Products.

Countries with the largest intake of milk, such as the USA and Sweden, have the highest rates of osteoporosis due to their high animal protein diets, a condition causing weakening and possible bone breakdown.' -Richard Schwartz, Ph.D. Research published in the Lancet Medical Journal identified a small group of patients in Norway with Chronic Fatigue Syndrome (CFS). They experienced significant change over four years by excluding milk and wheat from their diets. The reintroduction of these foods into their diets resulted in a significant rise in the cytokine levels of the patients, along with an increase in pain.

Milk further aggravates asthma due to its casein content, in addition to increasing cytokines. When another animal's protein is injected into the human body, the immune system may respond with an allergic reaction. Casein is a nutrient to the milk. Eating casein allows your body to produce histamines that contribute to excess mucus production.

Those with CFS and asthma aren't alone with their milk sensitivity. Studies suggest that a specific diary/mil protein is responsible for the development of diabetes, since patients produce antibodies to cow milk proteins, according to the New England Journal of Medicine, July 30th, 1992.

There's a lot of vices in Milk. The digestion of milk proteins, however weird it may sound, may produce an addictive substance that functions as endorphins, our own personal narcotics. Gluten and wheat can all be the same. These endorphins are capable of altering brain chemistry and of inducing addiction.

Gluten.

Gluten is a component of grains like wheat, rice, barley, and rye. In addition to being inflammatory, higher than the average number of people with autoimmune disorders have been reported to be allergic to gluten. We are recommending complete abstinence for at least one month to see if there will be benefits.

Research has also shown that wheat and corn can irritate Rheumatoid Arthritis patients and increase the production of cytokine in the colon and rectum of those with celiac disease.

Corn, Corn Syrup (Fructose), Corn Oil.

Corn has been named the leading cause of chronic food addiction in this century, in addition to fostering cytokines. To give you an understanding of how strong the addiction can be, all cigarettes made in the United States have contained added sugars, usually from corn, since World War I. Did you think corn syrup was selected by the cigarette companies for the great taste it brings to their products?

Corn syrup (fructose) is cheaper than cane sugar and twice as sweet. The average person ate 83 livres of fructose in 1994. Corn syrup causes an increase in lactic acid in the blood, particularly in people living with diabetes. Corn syrup fructose decreases copper absorption and increases the supply of minerals, two factors in autoimmunity. Also, fructose breaks down into a substance that weakens the natural anti-inflammatory molecules in your body. The body is not metabolizing fructose precisely the same as other sugars. More than any additional sugar, fructose transforms into fat. Indeed, corn fructose isn't the diabetic-friendly, and harmless sugar substitute claimed to be.

Studies have shown that maize can irritate patients with rheumatoid arthritis (RA), and the National Association of Fibromyalgia (NFA) recommends that maize should be avoided because it can aggravate fibromyalgia.

Note that if maize products can raise cytokine levels in those with RA and Fibromyalgia, cytokine levels can increase for anyone.

Sugar.

Americans consume 153 pounds of sugar a year on average. Refined white sugar makes it harder for your body to absorb vitamins and minerals, which are a major contributor to autoimmunity. Sugar also suppresses immune function, so that we are vulnerable to infection. Just eight tbsps of sugar, which is the sugar equivalent in less than one 12-ounce soda, will reduce the immune system's ability to destroy germs by up to 40%.

Sugar dehydrates the body like salt. Dehydration increases histamine, which can aggravate asthma and any other autoimmune disease because histamine enhances the development of cytokines. As suggested by the National Association for Fibromyalgia (NFA), sugars should be avoided because they can exacerbate the disorder. Sugar feeds on Lyme-causing bacteria and Candida yeast, which will be discussed later on. Eating sugar also induces an increase in insulin, leading to chronic inflammation.

Honey is sugar. It may be "all normal," but it's still sugar. This exceeds table sugar in calories and can be polluted with pesticides. Consuming delicious "completely natural" pesticide degustations isn't what you want to do.

The dietary supplement stevia is a good non-toxic alternative to sugar. Millions of people made use of stevia without reported side effects. Stevia sweetened goods constitute 41 percent of the consumed sweet substances market share in Japan.

Originally from Paraguay, Stevia is a herb. It is used by South Americans as a sweetener and for medicinal purposes. The herb is 30 to 100 times sweeter than sugar anywhere. Stevia doesn't affect most diabetic blood sugar levels. Stevia also does not feed the intestines with fungi as do sugars.

Stevia has a solid, sweet flavor that can overpower a recipe, so sparing use should be made of it. Because you use only such a small amount at a time, the recipes have to be changed due to the lack of volume. Stevia can often be purchased for bulk with useful inulin added to it. As well, stevia-sweetened cakes and cookies don't brown as much as their sugar-sweetened counterparts.

Flour / Processed Foods.

The next sentence will be one of the most painful ones in the novel, for you plain carbohydrate-lovers (addicts). If you want to rid yourself of cytokine inflammation, you have to give up processed food and junk food. They tend to be full of everything you're not supposed to eat. Many breakfast kinds of cereal, crackers, cookies, muffins, bread, and doughnuts are on this list.

White flour contains alloxan, that is the chemical used to make the flour appear white and clean. Alloxan destroys the pancreatic beta-cells, which produce insulin. It does this by causing free radical damage to the pancreatic Genome. Researchers believe that in these beta-cells, some people have weak resistance to free radicals. Alloxan is so active that it is used by researchers researching diabetes to infect laboratory animals with diabetes. Even though not everyone who eats white bread and foods has diabetes, the relation is clear: in those genetically prone to the disease, alloxan causes diabetes.

The Nightshade Family.

In the nightshade branch, vegetables include white potatoes, tomatoes, all peppers, cherries, tobacco, and aubergines. Research indicates that according to the National Fibromyalgia Association (NFA), these vegetables cause pain and inflammation in patients with arthritis and aggravate fibromyalgia. Not everybody will be immune to night-shade foods, though. The only way to know it is to avoid it and then put it back in your diet for weeks.

Everyone should actively avoid cigarettes, which is a poisonous member of the family Nightshade.

Coffee.

Coffee has had its medicinal purposes, although it is toxic. Among people with particular forms of asthma diagnosed, some caffeine-type chemicals in coffee have been proven effective in inducing bronchial dilatation. Even in the caffeine family, some modern-day asthma drugs are made from chemicals.

For those who use coffee as a natural asthma medication, it's important to remember that caffeine is a toxic chemical. The aim is to serve as an insecticide in plant life. In humans, caffeine suppresses the enzymes needed to make memory. It also increases blood sugar levels as well as insulin levels, increasing cytokine production, and aggravating diabetes.

Drinking decaffeinated coffee obviously isn't the solution either. People who drink more than one cup of decaffeinated coffee a day are considered much more likely to develop rheumatoid arthritis. The hypothesis is that chemically decaffeinated goods cause increased autoimmune risk. If you're going to drink decaffeinated coffee anyway, make sure it's using a non-chemical decaffeinating process, and the coffee has been grown organically. Too many man-made chemicals are introduced to those who do not drink organic coffee.

Alcohol.

The wine industry has persuaded America that a glass or two per day is good for your heart. Yet John Folts, Ph.D. at the University of Wisconsin, has done studies that show you would have to drink enough alcohol to be declared legally intoxicated to achieve such heart-healthy benefits. One safer option is grape juice. The study by Dr. Folt also found that only 10 to 12 ounces of violet grape juice were associated with lower blood clotting, hence a lower risk of heart disease than the red wine promises.

Alcohol breaks down to poison in the body called aldehyde, as well as being pro-inflammatory and addictive. Toxins are dangerous chemicals, which are not accepted as useful by the liver. Toxins invade cells and kill them, and attract germs. Aldehyde builds up in the brain, muscles, spinal cord, joints, and tissues where muscle fatigue, inflammation, and pain are caused.

How to Naturally Reduce Inflammation.

If we know it or not, we all experience regular inflammation, but few of us fully understand the crucial role that inflammation plays in our bodies and the havoc that it can bring upon us when it goes unchecked. Many see inflammation as the redness, fire, swelling, and pain we get from injury, and while that's real, it's just one kind of inflammation: it's acute. Inflammation is a natural process by itself, and without it, healing could not occur in the body. Acute inflammation is seen as a response of the body to injury, helping to heal and defend damaged tissue, and is at the core of protecting our bodies from illness and disease. This form of inflammation works to heal by bringing more nourishment and the operation of the immune system to the area that most needs it.

Where inflammation is harmful, and when it occurs as chronic inflammation is even deadly. As the name suggests, chronic inflammation describes an inflammation that lasts for weeks, months, and even years. It happens when the initial stimuli that contributed to acute inflammation continue, as the body interprets the stimulus while unresolved. Without the typical redness, fire, swelling, or discomfort that would usually be seen with acute inflammation, this type of inflammation can be insidious in nature, quietly destroying your tissues. Tissue damage is a classic sign of chronic inflammation, frequently causing the tissue to form fibrous or scar tissue that once existed at the repair site. The development of new blood vessels (or angiogenesis) is another common characteristic of chronic inflammation, which plays an essential role in many disease processes, including cancer.

Chronic inflammation was related to autoimmune disorders, allergic reactions, viral and bacterial infections, and a variety of other disease and disease processes, including:

- Asthma.
- Crohn's disease, multiple sclerosis, heart disease rheumatoid arthritis, diabetes, celiac disease, cancer, obesity, Alzheimer's, atherosclerosis, allergies.

And many other disorders (including others such as gastritis, endocarditis, tendonitis, etc.).

How to Naturally Reduce Inflammation:

Incorporate a high-quality daily multivitamin.

A poor quality vitamin is nothing more than a waste of your energy. They're indigestible, and they're going through your body without even ever doing anything useful to you. If you can find a liquid vitamin, then try it. These have 10 times higher absorption rates than tablets and capsules. If you already take a multivitamin, look at the folic acid and B vitamins you are using in the bottle. Such vitamins seem to play a role in reducing inflammation, although it is still unclear about how they do it in the medical community. Vitamin C, D, and E are other vitamins that have anti-inflammatory properties.

Try to add a little Mangosteen to your life.

A new medicinal fruit has been introduced in the United States in recent years, and it holds great promise for inflammation reduction, encouraging a healthy respiratory system and improving the immune system. Apparently, the fruit rind was used for thousands of years in folk medicine. Western medicine is beginning to give some serious attention to the little fruit because of its potent antioxidant and anti-inflammatory properties. The fruit is pulverized and added to the juice to create a nutritious beverage. A few ounces a day is all it takes for this little purple fruit to reap the benefits.

Ready. Set. GO!

In addition to naturally decreasing inflammation throughout the body, exercise has been shown to reduce the risk of heart disease, diabetes, and cancer, thereby reducing blood pressure, cholesterol, and improving mood and anxiety (lowering the risk of depression), and raising blood sugar levels, helping to improve body weight by reducing fat. If you're not used to exercising, simply walk each day slowly. Yoga and water aerobics are my two favorite low-impact forms of exercise— as you develop more stamina and strength, you will start to be more incorporated into your life. An important point to drive home is this: you do not have to cram yourself into a gym for exercise. Gardening, cooking, cycling, riding, and other forms of physical activity are something that we all need, and simply moving every day, together with eating a healthy diet, is the two most important things that you can do for your body.

Redefine Your Sweet Tooth.

Simple sugars, like those found in most processed foods, wreak havoc on our bodies, triggering an unexpected increase in our blood sugar levels, thereby increasing levels of insulin to counterbalance the spikes. It leads to a reduction in the role of the immune system, promotion of obesity, and an increase in inflammation increased levels of C-reactive protein, a marker of inflammation in the body. Eating complex carbohydrates, fruits, nuts, whole grains, seeds, vegetables, and healthy protein sources can help balance blood sugar levels while enhancing body satiety and reducing inflammatory processes. As a general rule, the more raw and unprocessed the food source is, the more the blood sugar levels are controlled.

Trim the FAT excess fat contained in fat cells (adipose tissue), by itself, allows inflammation and inflammatory processes to occur in the body.

However, these very inflammatory processes can lead to insulin-resistant type II diabetes as well as cortisol resistance, making it even more, harder to lose weight in those with obesity. Modification of diet, regular daily exercise, regulation of food portions, chewing your food twice as long as you would usually (eating at a slower pace), and getting family and friends support will help to overcome obesity once and for all, helping to prevent the many health conditions associated with obesity.

Break the habit

Apart from smoking being the number one cause of preventable disease and premature death, smoking has also been related to causing inflammation and rising C-reactive protein inflammatory markers, leading to heart disease, stroke, lung disease, and atherosclerosis. The body has immense potential for healing itself, and today quitting smoking will significantly enhance the chances of preventing the toxic and life-threatening effects that smokers face.

Get the carbohydrates and refined sugar out of your diet.

It's convenient, it's fast, it's easy, and it even tastes good at times, but it has to go. Refined foods do not have their place in a healthy diet. They just have to be reserved for special occasions and treatments. Not only are processed products filled with preservatives, colorants, and chemicals, but they can cause inflammation to flare up, leading to increased symptoms as well as allergies. The average person really only regularly eats around 20 foods. We prefer to be habit creatures and consume the foods that we love again and again. With just a little thinking, you can easily find healthy alternatives for your worst criminals. If you love lasagna, totally do not take it off your list forever. Put on ground turkey spelt or rice pasta. If you'd rather give up your chocolate than trust me, I can relate. Switch to dark chocolate; it is possible to switch to 60% cacao or higher. Check the ingredients for no high fructose corn syrups or funny stuff. You can hold your favorite foods with a little imagination and contemplation, quenching the discomfort and feeling fantastic.

Look out for foods that you may be susceptible to if left untreated these can cause chronic inflammation in the body.

The most common are wheat, sugar, milk, eggs, soy, and nuts. Eliminate them from your diet for a couple of weeks, and then put them back in one at a time. See if you notice any changes, such as headaches, foggy thinking, or bloating, to how you feel. If you consider a criminal, avoid it at all costs and look for alternatives to substitute it with. Seek soy or almond milk if you think you have a problem with the dairy.

Go out and play!

You have heard it a thousand times. I will tell you again. Stress is a killer and can undo all the hard work that you've done to control your inflammation. Just get rid of that stress in your life once and for all. Take some exercise and find something that you really like to do. Tennis, cycling, cooking, jumping dancing, pogo-sticking, it doesn't matter just turning your body in a way that you'll find fun doing daily. If it's a hassle and a burden, you're not actually adding to it to alleviate the stress. Breathe deeply, practice yoga, ponder meditation, forgive all those people who drive you nuts. Yeah, even that guy who cut off you on the freeway. If chronic stress is a real issue in your life, consider looking into biofeedback or counseling. Also, people with some kind of daily spiritual practice show lower stress rates. Look at counseling centers, synagogues, churches, and walking early in the morning once a week just to focus on how well you really do have it can make a profound difference in your stress levels and can help you regulate cortisol, the stress hormone.

Sleep it off.

An excellent strategy for reducing inflammation. Each night you need a proper amount of sleep to allow your body time to heal from the stresses of the day. Don't understate this. Napping reduces inflammation, as well. It is also a perfect excuse to turn off your phone in the middle of the day and decompress for 10 to 15 minutes. Remember, the more you sleep, the more hours before midnight. Going to bed by ten and waking at six will do your body better than going to bed by one and sleeping by eight.

Tea Time.

The beneficial effects of tea, specifically green and white tea, have become well known in popular culture. Still, it is worth highlighting the many benefits of tea, arising mainly from the polyphenol compounds they contain— helping to keep inflammation at bay through the potent antioxidants they contain. Clinically, tea has been shown to reduce the risk of cancer, heart disease, diabetes, high cholesterol, atherosclerosis, bowel disease, and hepatic disease (to name a few), thus assisting with weight loss and the symptoms of arthritis (and other inflammatory diseases). Realize also that all non-herbal teas contain these beneficial polyphenol compounds, from green tea to black tea, but the darker the tea, the more fermentation, and processing has occurred, and the more caffeine is present, so selecting a white tea or green tea will give you more of these beneficial compounds.

Find Your Inner Peace.

Stress is an absolute killer—-we know that much, yet the degree to which stress kills is astounding. Stress has been linked to heart disease, stroke, high cholesterol, depression, diabetes, colds, kidney disease, asthma, ulcers, and cancer (to name but a few), and it has been shown to increase C-reactive protein, causing inflammation in the body. Many stress reduction techniques include: daily exercise, meditation and praying to clear the mind, talking to loved ones or a therapist, yoga and tai chi (or qi gong), taking time to spend with family and friends, laughing regularly and, as Dr. Mercola also recommends, the technique of emotional liberation (an example of EFT can be found here), which I use and endorse personally. We find that daily changes in our clinic have helped our patients cope with the side effects of stress, thus helping to manage stress.

The Good Fat.

As the name suggests, essential fatty acids are important fats for our survival— our bodies are unable to produce them, so we need to get these fats from our diets. Sadly, the standard American diet contains 14 to 25 times more omega-6 fats than omega-3, although the omega-3 to omega-6 ratio should be closer to 1:1. There are numerous conditions associated with insufficient intake of omega-3 fat, ranging from heart disease and mood disorders such as ADHD and schizophrenia to rheumatoid arthritis and lupus. In the end, this is we need to make a conscious effort every day to ensure that we get our omega-3 fats to help drive down inflammation in the body and protect our brain, heart, and neural tissue. Good sources of omega-3 fats can be found in many seeds and nuts, such as walnuts and flax seeds, as well as wild fish species, particularly wild salmon and krill or cod liver oil, as well as eggs. It is important to distinguish between farmed salmon and wild-caught salmon— they are not the same and provide vastly different nutrient levels that our bodies need. Also, with increased pollution, making sure to buy fish that contains the lowest levels of heavy metals, such as mercury, has become very important.

Eat more wild fish/seafood, and increase your usual fruit and vegetable intake.

I know that sounds very easy, but it's true. Eating more fruits and vegetables, the dark greens mainly will dramatically reduce your body's inflammation. Meals rich in brightly colored vegetables contain natural anti-inflammatory properties and fiber. Try selecting wild varieties over farm-raised when considering seafood if you have to choose for an organic farm-raised look. Salmon is the best bet you can make but stick to the wild variation. Farm-raised salmon fed a rich cornmeal diet that can help improve inflammation. Try to stick to Pacific fish and avoid the Atlantic varieties that contain higher mercury and PCB levels.

Get those essential fatty acids into your diet (EFA's).

One of the simplest ways to control chronic inflammation is by adding omega-3 fatty acids to your diet, and, luckily, it's fast. Adding a few nuts and seeds to your diet can boost your omega-3s intact. Walnuts, ground flaxseed, and pumpkin and sesame seeds are the best choices. Some good sources for the omega-3s are avocados and darkly leafy greens. Mixing a salad with a spoonful of grapeseed oil will ensure you get your regular omega-3 dose. You can also take a supplement for the fish oil. Look for products containing wild fish oil and low mercury levels. If you're a vegetarian, you can try flaxseed oil or algal sources.

Healthy Herbs (and Spices!).

In many of our prescription pain drugs, cox-II inhibitors are prevalent and were present in Vioxx, the drug that was eventually pulled out of the market for its connection to heart attack and stroke. Cox-II inhibitors are also naturally present in many medicines, with much lower efficacy than prescription drugs and with fewer side effects, working to reduce inflammation in the body. Most herbs have been used to model the medicines that we use today. In the case of aspirin, it was initially being based on white willow bark that contains salicin (similar to, but less potent than the synthetic aspirin acetylsalicylic acid). Herbs such as turmeric (curcumin), white willow bark, ginger, devil's claw, Boswellia, and hops have all been shown to decrease inflammation, providing benefits, especially for arthritis sufferers naturally. While not a plant, Bromelain, a protein-digestive enzyme contained in pineapple, has also proven effective with inflammation and treating body injury. Consider cooking more meals at home using new, organic herbs and spices, as many contain beneficial compounds that improve the innate ability of our body to heal itself naturally.

Non-chemical.

This year, both the Environmental Working Group and the President's Cancer Panel issued reports describing the dangers of certain chemicals, contaminants, and pollutants that pose specific threats to our safety. Conditions associated with environmental contaminants and chemicals are extensive but usually include: defects in the endocrine and nervous system, asthma, cancer, inflammation of the skin, eye and lung, ADHD, and a weakened immune system. The studies concluded that people should buy organically wherever possible, drink filtered water, be mindful of contaminants to the atmosphere (such as radon), and make efforts to avoid other chemicals in the households.

Take The Taste Buds for a Mediterranean Trip.

The Mediterranean diet has long been proven effective in helping prevent heart disease, cancer, Alzheimer's disease, obesity, and type II diabetes, among the many other health benefits it promotes. The diet focuses on consuming plenty of fresh, ideally locally grown fruits, vegetables, nuts, and seeds, whole grains, and nutrient-healthy oils (like olive oil) on a daily basis while adding less-healthy oils. Red meat is eaten sparingly in favor of fish, chicken, and eggs— all of which are consumed in much fewer amounts than we usually eat in the standard American diet. Considering your diet, take into account the patterns around us, remembering that the way we do things now is not the way we've always done things and that obesity, type II diabetes, heart disease, cancer, etc. Americans consumed 144 pounds of meat In 1950 (on average) per human per year. Jump ahead to 2007, and we see that the average American now consumes nearly 222 pounds of meat per year—-an astounding 78 pounds more meat per person per year in just 57 years! The change starts with you.

Treating Inflammation At The Source.

Pulsed electromagnetic fields (PEMF's) were used to treat almost any possible human disease or illness, including many inflammatory conditions like arthritis or psoriasis. PEMF therapy was associated with a reduction of pain and improved healing. PEMF's exert these effects by, among other biological actions, controlling processes involving inflammation and autoimmune diseases.

Inflammation is a series of physiological processes instigated by the body to repair cellular damage in healthy blood-supplied tissues and return the tissue to its normal function. Typical signs and symptoms of inflammation include:

Redness caused by increased blood flow, the heat generated by the leukocyte metabolism and macrophages recruited to the damaged site, swelling due to edema, and pain caused by the development of pro-inflammatory prostaglandins.

This inflammation is the net result of a cascade of biological processes, produced and assisted by the interaction of several types of immune cells, including lymphocytes, macrophages, and neutrophils, with other types of cells, such as fibroblasts, endothelial cells, and vascular smooth muscle cells, playing a regulatory role in the cascade.

Chronic inflammation vs. acute.

Although inflammation is a natural as well as beneficial process, its severity may become abnormally elevated during the initial acute phase, and often lasts longer than necessary, leading to chronic inflammation. Chronic inflammation is associated with one or more aspects of the immune system dysfunction and leads to recurrent tissue damage in diseases such as tendinitis, arthritis, or psoriasis. Chronic inflammation, among many other forms of sickness, is also a cause of cancer and Alzheimer's disease.

Inflammation Mechanics.

Numerous targets for therapies aimed at regulating inflammation in the acute phase and preventing progression to chronic inflammation are provided by the different cell types and metabolic pathways that produce inflammation. Many causes can cause inflammation, and it is essential to know and understand the nature of the cause when developing therapeutic strategies. Early penetration of the infected tissues by polymorphonuclear neutrophils (PMNs), a type of white blood cell, is accompanied in bacterial infections by the arrival of T cells, an event required to kill bacteria. Eliminating T cells in this situation will slow or stop the healing. T cells are less important for repairing tissue damage in trauma-induced injury and can be harmful if present for long periods.

In this case, early removal of T cells in the acute phase of inflammation may mitigate the undesirable inflammatory effects, improve healing, and reduce the risk of chronic inflammatory disease. Persistence of the disease state in chronic inflammatory disorders such as rheumatoid arthritis, psoriasis, and chronic tendinitis depends on the involvement of T cells. Here, a beneficial treatment strategy for these and related chronic conditions would be to kill T cells. The T-cells are a primary inflammatory cascade regulator. Research has shown that PEMF's can cause sufficient T lymphocyte death through actions on T cell membranes and main cell enzymes. For example, PEMFs have been shown to influence ion flow through specific channels of the cell membrane, including those for sodium, potassium, and calcium, which have a positive effect on these enzymes. Such appropriate results help to reduce chronic inflammation.

Homeostasis And Cells Out Of Balance.

Healthy cells usually are not affected by magnetic fields. Compromised cells, or meta-stable cells, have a higher chance of being affected. It suggests that PEMFs have a greater impact in conditions where tissue or cell imbalances, i.e., where disease or chronic inflammation occurs. Where homeostasis is robust in the body, PEMF's are unlikely to have effects, notably weaker PEMF's. For instance, activation of the T cell receptor, as occurs with PPEMF's, often stimulates different processes in the cell that return to normal levels within five minutes of removing the activating signal.

Inflammation Reduction By PEMF's.

There are significant changes in other white blood cells called lymphocytes, both from low intensity, low-frequency PEMF, and even DC / permanent magnetic fields. PEMF communicates in often unexpected ways with the cellular networks, which means that increasing frequency and/or intensity does not always result in a one-to-one shift in the intensity of reaction. The growth of PEMF inhibits and the natural death of unwanted lymphocytes that decreases inflammation. Following EMF therapy, the EMF suppression of lymphocytes and then inflammatory processes seem to be most apparent 48 to 72 hours, and then the EMF effect tends to be gone. This suggests PEMF's effects can work well with other natural treatments.

The use of EMF for inflammation needs to be tailored so that exposure results in long-lasting, therapeutically relevant results. Higher frequency fields that are modulated by pulse-bursts tend to be much more powerful than other frequency signals, and thus Servings better therapeutic effects. Although particular types of signals may be most effective, various types of magnetic stimulation are often seen as having a positive response. Similar results tend to have on lymphocytes using pulsed bone healing fields and fields in the direction of the sinusoidal power line. Pulsed PEMF's with 5-25 MilliTesla intensities did not have any effect on normal T cells. This means that normal lymphocytes do not get any apparent damage.

Inflammatory T cells form interleukin-2(IL-2), which stimulates T cell growth. The desired early removal of these chronic inflammatory cells improves when the IL-2 levels are high enough. Cells exposed to pulsed PEMFs can account for up to a triple increase in IL-2. EMF intensity gaps appear to exist, but these have not been well described. Frequency windows have been shown to differ across different tissue cell types within the body. The frequency ranges for bone cells tend to be relatively narrow. The frequency ranges tend to be larger for the lymphocytes. Also, 5-100 hertz, 0.15 mT signals modulate the calcium flux in the lymphocytes, with the greatest effect being 50 Hz PEMF. Frequency fields were also found to have an operation, in conjunction with parallel static magnetic fields. Knowing that PEMF affects all lymphocytes, including B cells and T cells and other lymphoid cell lines in humans, is essential.

EMF therapy targets specific cells that are meta-stable as a result of disease or other ongoing therapies. Therefore, PEMF's can be an effective cellular therapy in many diseases, including cancer, psoriasis, wound healing, and bacterial infections due to their chronic inflammation reduction effects. PEMF's mustn't affect normal homeostatically stable cells, allowing other therapies to be more successful without significant increases in side effects. Cells are characteristically retained in meta-stable states in chronic inflammatory diseases, as a consequence of cytokine secretions and other related stressors. PEMF's can act as a stand-alone anti-inflammatory therapy in such cases. Even the slow, low-frequency PEMF induces apoptosis in activated T cells, reducing chronic inflammation without having an adverse effect on acute inflammation.

Inflammation-Eating Food That Is Anti-Inflammatory.

Are there really diets that can help reduce inflammation? Are they working? Scientists found there is, in part, a connection between what we consume and inflammation. Researchers have even found some food compounds that can decrease inflammation and others that stimulate it. There's still much to learn about how diet and inflammation interact, and study is not yet at the stage where it's possible to identify specific foods or food groups as beneficial to people with arthritis. We're trying to get a clearer picture of how it will minimize inflammation in the right way to eat.

And why are we so concerned with inflammation? Inflammation is the normal protection of the body against diseases and injuries. When something goes wrong, the immune system of the body goes to work to inflammate the region that helps to get rid of the invader or repair the wound. Inflammation can cause pain, redness, swelling, and warmth, but as soon as the problem is solved, this goes away. The inflammation is healthy.

Then we have chronic inflammation, the sort that people with rheumatoid arthritis (RA), lupus, psoriatic arthritis, and other "inflammatory" arthritis are familiar with. Some kind of chronic inflammation that won't go away is all the types of arthritis listed above are an immune system disorder that causes inflammation and then doesn't know when to shut down. Inflammatory arthritis, chronic inflammation can have severe consequences, lifelong injury and tissue damage can be one if it is not adequately treated. Inflammation was linked with several other medical conditions.

It has been shown that inflammation leads to atherosclerosis, which is when fat builds up on the lining of the arteries, raising the risk of heart attacks. Inside the blood of people with heart disease, too, high levels of inflammation proteins were found. Inflammation was also associated with obesity, diabetes, asthma, depression, and even cancer and Alzheimer's disease. Scientists think a persistent degree of inflammation can have a number of adverse effects in the body, even if the level is low. Research shows that diet can reduce inflammation; an inflammation-lowering diet can, in principle, affect a wide range of conditions of health.

Scientists have been looking for clues in our early ancestors ' eating habits to figure out which foods could help us the most. They agree that these patterns are more in line with the way the body absorbs and uses what we eat and drink. The diet of our ancestors was wild lean meats (venison or boar) and wild plants (green leafy vegetables, fruit, nuts, and berries). Until the agricultural revolution (about 10,000 yrs ago), there had been no cereal grains. There was a minimal amount of dairy and no processed or refined food. Our diets are usually high in meat, saturated (or bad) fats, and processed foods, and minimal exercise is needed. Nearby or as far away as our screen and a click of a mouse is virtually all we eat.

Our diet and lifestyles with how our bodies are made from the inside out are way out of whack. Although our genetic make-up has changed very little since we began, our diet and habits have changed a lot, and over the last 50 to 100 years, the changes have got worse. Our genes didn't have the opportunity to adapt.

We don't give our bodies the right type of fuel; it's like we think of our bodies as jet plane engines when they're like the engine in the very first planes instead. There are some foods that we put into our bodies, particularly because we eat too much of them, which are badly affecting our health.

Our diets have attracted attention with two foods, omega-3 fatty acids and omega-6 fatty acids have been a part of our diets for many years. For just about all of our many cells, they are components and are necessary for normal growth and development. Both of those acids play an inflammatory role. In some of the studies, it has been found that certain sources of omega 3, in particular, help minimize the inflammatory cycle and that it will be increased by the omega 6.

Now that's the question; the average American eats about 15 times more omega 6's on average than the omega 3's. While the ate omega 6's and omega 3's of our very early ancestor are in equal proportion, and it is assumed that this is what helped balance their ability to turn on and off inflammation. It is known that the deficiency of omega 3 and omega 6's in our diets leads to the excess inflammation of our bodies.

So why do we eat so many of the omega 6's now? Vegetable oils, like corn oil, safflower oil, cotton oil, sunflower oil, soybean oil, and the products made from them, such as margarine, are filled with omega 6's. Even those oils are made of many of the refined snack foods that are so readily available today. Based on the best knowledge of the time, vegetable oils such as those mentioned above were used in place of foods with saturated fats such as butter and lard. It looks like the effects of that advice may have led to increased omega 6 intake and thus created an imbalance of omega 3's and omega 6's.

Omega 6's can be found in other common foods, including meats and egg yolks. Omega 6 that is found in meat, is the fatty acids that derive from animals fed with grain such as goats, lambs, pigs, and chickens. Like their grass-fed counterparts, which contain less of those fatty acids, most of the meat sold in America is fed on corn. Wild game like venison and boar are lower in omega 6's and fat and higher in omega 3's than the meat from the supermarkets we're shopping for.

Omega 3s can be found in animal and plant milk. The bodies can more easily convert omega 3s from animal sources into anti-inflammatory compounds from plant sources than the omega 3s. Plant foods contain hundreds of other safe compounds, many of which are anti-inflammatory, so don't cut them all off together.

Some foods are high in omega-3s and include fatty fish, especially cold-water fish. Of course, everyone knows about salmon, but you knew that in mackerel, anchovies, sardines, herring, striped bass, and bluefish, you could also find omega 3s. Wild fish are also widely known to be better sources of omega 3s than those produced by the farms. You can buy eggs that are filled with omega 3 oils, too. In plants, which are leafy greens (like kale, Swiss chard, and spinach), as well as flaxseed, wheat germ, walnuts, and their oils, there are several excellent sources of omega-3s.

You can as well get omega 3s in supplements (often as fish oil); in some instances, this source has proven beneficial. Before taking a fish oil supplement, you should take it with your doctor because it can interfere with some drugs and may increase the risk of bleeding under certain circumstances. I'm taking a prescription omega-3 supplement because my doctor told me that those you get in a pharmacy or health food store are not pure; they have other additives that don't help at all. Certain fats leading to clogged arteries, the "poor" or saturated fats contained in meats and high-fat dairy products, are called pro-inflammatory fats.

Trans fats are also relatively new to the cause of heart disease. Such Trans fats can be present in packaged convenience foods and snacks and can be identified by reading the label. These can be discerned as partially hydrogenated oils, mostly soybean oil or cotton oil. Yet naturally, they can also occur in small amounts in animal feed. The theory is that they contribute to our bodies' pro-inflammatory behaviors, and the quantities that we eat today are overwhelming.

Antioxidants are substances that prevent inflammation from overtaking our bodies, which causes "free radicals." Plant foods, including fruit, vegetables (including beans), nuts, and seeds, carry high concentrations of antioxidants. Extra virgin olive oil and walnut oil are powerful antioxidant sources, too. Such ingredients have long been considered the fundamentals of good health and can be found in vivid and vibrant pigments in fruits and vegetables. From green vegetables, particularly leafy ones, to low-starch vegetables like broccoli and cauliflower, to berries, tomatoes, brightly colored orange, yellow fruits, and vegetables, the more colorful the plant is, the better they are for you.

I bet you wonder what Arthritis has to do with that. Okay, some research has been done on diet and arthritis, concentrating mostly on RA. There was a study that analyzed a lot of other diets and RA research and found diets rich in omega 3's had some effect on reducing RA symptoms. Another study published in 2008 found that omega 6 fatty acids and omega 3 fatty acids are consumed in a ratio of 3 or 2 to 1 (a small ratio relative to the 15-1 ratio in the diet of most people) decreased inflammation in people with RA. There was also a study that found taking omega 3 may also allow humans to reduce their use of no steroidal anti-inflammatory drugs (NSAIDs), such as ibuprofen (Advil, Motrin) and naproxen (Aleve). But these and other researchers do not provide sufficient evidence to prove that there is any specific anti-inflammatory diet that can really affect the symptoms of arthritis. It doesn't mean the diets are harmful; it just means there may come a day when studies will prove its benefits. In the future, diet, along with exercise and medicine, can be considered one of many resources that can be used to reduce the symptoms of arthritis.

We do not have to absolutely return to the caveman to eat the anti-inflammatory way of benefiting from the anti-inflammatory diet. Only eating a healthy diet prescribed today is well on its way. Our main strategy should be to match the number of modern-day foods with old-fashioned foods, which were rich in food-reducing inflammation. All we need to do is replace foods rich in omega 6 with foods rich in omega 3, cut down on how much meat and poultry we consume while consuming oily fish a few days a week and add more varieties of colorful fruits and vegetables. While whole grains were not part of the diet of our early ancestors, they should be included in our diet. Make sure it is whole grains and not refined grains since they contain many beneficial nutrients and compounds that are inflammatory. Researchers found that consuming plenty of foods high in sugar and white flour can promote inflammation, although more study is needed on the issue.

The amount of knowledge we have about how the body works and how the ate of our ancestors helps to validate the adage: "You are what you eat." But we need to learn more before we can recommend any anti-inflammatory diet. Our genetic makeup and the nature of our health condition will decide the benefits we derive from an anti-inflammatory diet, and there is sadly uncertainty that there will be one diet that suits all of us.

Whether we eat or not eat is also just a small part of the entire story. We're not as physically active as our ancestors and have their own anti-inflammatory effects on physical activity. Our ancestors have also been much leaner than we are, and body fat is active tissue that can produce compounds causing inflammation.

Anti-inflammatory eating is a way to choose foods which are more in line with what the body needs. By going back to our roots, we will achieve a more balanced diet. Looking at the Bible people's lifestyle, you'll find that they were more physical, like our caveman ancestors, and their diets were much the same items as our caveman ancestors were. They had no choice but to walk everywhere they needed to go, nothing like cars or trucks. While today we have it better, our health has suffered greatly from this.

Chapter 2: Anti-Inflammatory Diet.

In recent years anti-inflammatory diets have become common. The suggested foods are characteristic of a Mediterranean diet and include consuming more fresh fruits fish, and vegetables, and healthy fats, eating small quantities of nuts, eating very little red meat, and drinking moderate red wine. Like the Mediterranean diet, the ideals of an anti-inflammatory diet are healthy ones, and according to the Mayo Clinic, the strategy is nutritionally sound.

"Anti-inflammatory food ingredients, such as omega-3 fats, protect the body from potential inflammatory damage," said Ximena Jimenez, a Miami-based nutritionist and Academy of Nutrition and Dietetics spokesperson.

An anti-inflammatory diet also ensures that foods that can cause inflammation are kept away. According to the University of Wisconsin, it's best to minimize the number of foods you eat high in saturated and trans fats, like red meats, dairy products, and foods that contain partially hydrogenated oils. Therefore, reduce sugar foods and refined carbohydrates, including white rice and bread. Or cut back on the use of omega-6 fatty acids found in cooking oils or margarine, such as corn, safflower, and sunflower oils.

Benefits of an Anti-Inflammatory Diet.

Inflammation quickly becomes the next major medical discovery. People with obesity have trouble with inflammation. Diabetes, arthritis, and asthma all contribute to inflammation in the body. Not to mention the link to various heart conditions and cancers. Reducing the body's inflammation with an anti-inflammation diet will cause an immediate improvement in how you feel, not to mention the long-term health and wellbeing benefits of the dietary change.

The first step in following an anti-inflammatory diet is to consider the body's effects on food. The food contains nutrition and the body needs vitamins to survive. The idea of eating to live not to eat is a huge push for the culture in weight loss, but this idea should not only be pursued when a few pounds need to be lost. Many foods have high concentrations of antioxidants and natural anti-inflammatory nutrients, which may reduce inflammatory effects on the body. It is these foods that are at the heart of the anti-inflammatory diet.

The Omega 3 Function and Other Fatty Acids.

Many foods that contain oil contain fatty acids. Fish like salmon and sardines are the best natural choice. Omega 6 fatty acids are, however, dominant over Omega 3s in western diets. This is because common foods are high in Omega 6 fatty acids, such as chicken, turkey, eggs, nuts, and vegetable oils. However, what people don't realize is that for optimum health and anti-inflammatory action, these fatty acids must be balanced with Omega 3s. Omega 6s are 10 times more than Omega 3s in most western diets. Many diets take up as much as 30 times as much. The optimum ratio for every 1 part Omega 3 is 4 parts Omega 6.

Increasing Omega 3 fatty acids in the diet can minimize inflammation in the body and thus reduce the health and general wellbeing impact of this disorder. Foods that are high in Omega 3s contain fish oil, kiwi, black raspberry, and many different nuts. Flaxseeds are the most readily available source of Omega 3s. Many people mistake fish oils for the best source, but flaxseed oils appear to have the Omega 3s that are most readily available to promote absorption in the body. Flaxseed oils contain approximately 55 percent ALA (alpha-linolenic acid), an Omega 3 fatty acid.

Fatty Meats Be Gone.

The reduction of fatty meats is another simple change to reduce inflammation in the body. Red meat is the worst of all foods for an inflammation sufferer. It is an excellent option to choose a leaner cut or slimmer substitute. Bison and venison are two choices that appear to have less fat in them. Grass-fed cows have less inflammatory effects on the body, too. All lean options for reducing inflammation are fish, lean chicken, turkey, soybeans, tofu, and soy milk. But in Omega 6s, some of those meats tend to be higher. Try cooking these meats in olive oil or adding flaxseed oil to the final dish to raise Omega 3s to reduce the fatty acid imbalance, which may increase inflammation.

The Danger of Processed Foods.

Refined starch is the worst food to eat while suffering from inflammations. Such foods provide very little nutritional value and should be replaced with alternatives to whole grain. All meal is wheat-based, but the refined meal is stripped of wholesome grain wholesomeness and bleached. What's left are empty calories that will undoubtedly fill the body even more. It can make a big difference in how your body reacts to your diet by simply replacing white bread with whole-grain bread and white flour with whole wheat flour, which is unbleached.

Foods that Affect Your Inflammatory Diet.

You chose to take back your life and health and follow an anti-inflammatory diet. Most people make the same choice to counter the effects of obesity, diabetes, arthritis, and other disorders of inflammation. As with any dietary change, the control once assumed over the foods eaten will grow lax after a period of time. The same foods also creep back into the diet and reduce the anti-inflammatory diet's effectiveness. These include packaged foods, blends of butter, and margarine. The remaining common factors are the reduction of protein and water intake.

Packaged food is just plain bad for your body. These foods also contain enough sodium and healthy fat for a whole day. Although popping a meal in the microwave two or three times a week may seem innocuous, the effect can be dramatic. Prepackaged meals range between 700 and 1000 calories each. Only three meals a week can contribute an extra 3000 calories to the diet, not to mention the fat and sodium rises. High-fat meals induce inflammation in the body for hours after intake and can result in weight gain that causes further inflammation.

On the budget, oil blends are better than the plain olive oil. Nonetheless, these blends can contain oils that contain trans fats. Such fats are unhealthy and should not be consumed in the diet at ALL. Saving a bit of money on the front side will negate your healthy, back-side, anti-inflammatory diet choices.

Margarine is cheaper than butter, which contains fewer calories. Many people even think eating pure butter will lead to an increase in cholesterol levels that can lead to stroke. NOT that is the case. Those who choose to consume very low carbohydrate diets, which often involve high doses of butter, measure lower cholesterol numbers than their peers consuming margarine or low fat.

Protein is costly, and lean protein is capable of breaking the budget. When money is tight, it may seem like a safe option to buy the fatty burger to replace the 93/7 lean beef, which was part of your anti-inflammatory diet. Fatty red meat is associated with increased cancer risk and induces inflammation in the body. Instead, try to replace the burger, which will all beans together.

Water is life's fluid and drinking water is the best choice for improving overall health and reducing inflammation. Most people start an anti-inflammatory diet by taking half a gallon or more of water a day. Over time, the lax activity can result in an increased intake of caffeine and a decreased intake of water. Caffeine is associated with inflammation and can make the anti-inflammatory diet less effective in reducing inflammation.

The anti-inflammatory diet is not about exclusively banning all foods, which could increase inflammation. Deprivation is the number one reason people are scrapping new diets and going back to old eating habits. Instead of depriving people, seek healthier alternatives, or actually reduce the number of times they eat prepackaged foods, fat red meats, and trans-fat-based oils. It's not the problem, once in a while. It is when this happens every week or every day once in a while that inflammation will return even if you believe you are adopting an anti-inflammatory diet.

The Biggest Anti-Inflammatory Diet Challenges.

Everybody wants to feel better and live healthier. One of the best ways to achieve this is by transitioning to an anti-inflammatory diet from a traditional western diet. Making the shift is simple, but as a diet plan, it can be difficult to stick to the changes in food and watch what you eat.

Fast Food and Your Inflammation.

Fast food is an incredible impediment to an anti-inflammatory diet. Foods high in fat tend to increase inflammatory substances in the body 3-4 hours after the meal. If the same number of calories is consumed as fresh fruits, vegetables, and lean meats in one fast-food sitting, the effect will not occur. It is also possible to increase free radicals, cell killers that exacerbate inflammatory problems after eating fast food by 175 percent.

The Alternative-A substitute, anti-inflammatory diet, is the best alternative to fast food. Take into consideration the McDonald's Big Mac. You can make this sandwich from lean ground turkey and a whole grain bun. The "unique" sauce can be combined with lower ketchup of carbohydrates, mayonnaise of olive oil, and relish free of sugar. The effect is a savory alternative with a considerably lower fat count.

Red Meat, Milk, and Your Inflammation.

Science has long struggled to equate red meat to certain forms of cancer. Little did they know the work would lead to a link between this common protein and inflammation in the dinner. Researchers believe that the body behaves defensively on certain chemical elements of red meat and milk. If the body thinks that these are different things, then the immune system will kick in, and inflammation will occur. Imagine once a day eating red meat and drinking two or three glasses of milk. The body will live in a state of persistent or chronic inflammation that could potentially cause health problems.

Alternative-Lean meat, beef, and fish all form part of a healthy diet. Beef is a fantastic source of iron, so it is not a requirement to remove it. But it is important for good health to choose the slimmest of cuts. Lean proteins and beans represent the finest meats.

Your Inflammation And Trans Fats.

Trans fatty acid is a secret cause of inflammation of the body. Although many people know a little about this kind of fat, few understand the effects on the body. Fast food, baked goods, prepackaged food, and margarine are often strong trans fat sources. Those fats can increase the risk of coronary artery disease, insulin resistance, diabetes, and heart failure after entering the body. Increased risk of stroke is also common because of abnormally high lipid levels. Although many foods claim to be trans fat-free, that is not the whole reality. These products can contain up to 0.5 grams of trans fats per serving according to the labeling guidelines, and still mark the product as "trans-fat-free." Such small amounts, if the diet is high in processed food, margarine, and baked goods, will add up over time.

The alternative-Natural fats such as whole butter and olive oil do not contain trans fats. A good first step is to choose these in place of hydrogenated oils and margarine. When it comes to foods cooked in trans fat, there's no alternative but to remove all of these together from the diet. Many people choose to take an anti-inflammatory diet by baking their own snacks and home-style "fast-food" meals.

Chapter 3: Anti-Inflammatory Diet Recipes.

Breakfast And Brunch.

Green Shakshuka

Prep: 20 min
Cook: 25 min
Total: 55 min
4 servings

Ingredients

- 2 tablespoons extra-virgin olive oil
- 1 onion, minced
- 2 garlic cloves, minced
- 1 jalapeño, seeded and minced
- 1 pound spinach (thawed if frozen)
- 1 teaspoon dried cumin
- ¾ teaspoon coriander
- Salt and freshly ground black pepper
- 2 tablespoons harissa
- ½ cup vegetable broth
- 8 large eggs
- Chopped fresh parsley, as needed for serving
- Chopped fresh cilantro, as needed for serving
- Red-pepper flakes, as needed for serving

Instructions

- Preheat the oven to 350 ° F.

- Heat the olive oil inside a large, oven-safe skillet, over medium heat. Attach the onion and sauté for 4 to 5 minutes, until tender. Stir in the garlic and jalapeño, then sauté 1 minute more until fragrant.

- Add the spinach and cook until fully wilted if fresh, 4 to 5 minutes or 1 to 2 minutes if thawed from frozen, until heated through.

- Season with cumin, pepper, coriander, salt, and harissa. Cook for approximately 1 minute, until fragrant.

- Switch the mixture to a food processor bowl or a blender and puree until it is coarse. Connect the broth and purée until smooth and thick.

- Wipe the skillet out and dust it with nonstick cooking spray. Pour the spinach mixture into the pan back and make eight circular wells using a wooden spoon.

- Crack the eggs in the pipes, softly. Switch the skillet to the oven and cook for 20 to 25 minutes until the egg whites are set fully, but the yolks are still a little jiggly.

- Sprinkle with parsley, cilantro, and red pepper flakes on the shakshuka, to taste. Serve straight away.

Nutrition Info

251 calories
17g fat
10g carbs
17g protein
3g sugars

5-Minute Golden Milk

Creamy, simple golden milk with dairy-free milk, ginger, coconut oil, and turmeric. Sweetened, of course, amazingly good, and so delicious. Total time: only five minutes!

Prep Time 1 minute
Cook Time 4 minutes
Total Time 5 minutes
Servings: (glasses)

Ingredients

- 1 1/2 cps light coconut milk (canned is best; also carton works too)
- 1 1/2 cps unsweetened plain almond milk
- 1 1/2 teasp ground turmeric
- 1/4 teasp ground ginger
- 1 whole cinnamon stick (or 1/4 tsp ground cinnamon)
- 1 Tbsp coconut oil
- 1 pinch ground black pepper
- Sweetener of choice (i.e., coconut sugar, maple syrup, or stevia to taste)

Instructions

- Add coconut milk, ground turmeric, almond milk, ground ginger, cinnamon stick, coconut oil, black pepper and preferred sweetener to a small casserole (I usually add 1 Tbsp (15 ml) maple syrup/quantity as the original recipe is written/alter if the batch size changes).
- Whisk to mix over medium heat and warm up. Heat to the touch until hot but do not boil-about 4 minutes-whisking regularly.
- Turn off heat and taste to make flavor change. For strong spice + flavor, add more sweetener to taste, or more turmeric or ginger.
- Serve straight away, break between two glasses, and leave the cinnamon stick behind. Best when fresh, although the leftovers can be kept 2-3 days in the refrigerator. Reheat up to temperature on the stovetop or microwave.

Nutrition Info

Calories: 205
Fat: 19.5g
Saturated fat: 15.1g
Sodium: 161mg
Carbohydrates: 8.9g
Fiber: 1.1g
Protein: 3.2g

Steel Cut Oats With Kefir And Berries

Cook time: 30 mins

Serves: 4

Ingredients

For the oats:

- 1 cup steel-cut oats
- 3 cups water
- pinch of salt

For topping Optional:

- fresh or frozen fruit/berries
- a handful of sliced almonds, hemp seeds, pepitas, or other nuts/seeds
- unsweetened kefir, homemade/store-bought
- a drizzle of maple syrup, sprinkling of coconut sugar, a few drops of stevia, or any other sweetener you like, to taste

Instructions

- Add/place the oats in a small saucepan and over medium-high heat. Make the pan toast, often stir or shake, for 2-3 minutes.
- Adding the water and bring to a boil. Reduce heat to a cooker and let it cook for about 25 minutes, or until the oats are soft enough to satisfy you. (The oats will thicken as they cool — if you want a little bit more porridgy, add a splash of water or any milk or dairy-free alternative.) Serve with berries, nuts/seeds (or a handful of granola),

a splash of kefir, and any sweetener you like, to taste. Dig in!

Rhubarb, apple + ginger muffin recipe

8 servings

Ingredients

- 1/2 teaspoon ground cinnamon
- 1/2 teaspoon ground ginger
- a good pinch fine sea salt
- 1/2 cup almond meal (ground almonds)
- 1/4 cup unrefined raw sugar
- 2 tbspoons finely chopped crystallized ginger
- 1 tbspoon ground linseed meal
- 1/2 cup buckwheat flour
- 1/4 cup fine brown rice flour
- 1/4 cup (60ml) olive oil
- 1 large free-range egg
- 1 teaspoon vanilla extract
- 2 tablespoons organic cornflour or true arrowroot
- 2 teaspoons gluten-free baking powder
- 1 cup finely sliced rhubarb
- 1 small apple, peeled, and finely diced
- 95ml (1/3 cup + 1 tbspoon) rice or almond milk

Instructions

- Pre-heat the oven to 180C/350C. Grease or line 8 1/3 cup (80ml) cup muffin tins with paper case cap.

- In a medium bowl, put the almond meal, ginger, sugar, and linseed. Sieve over baking powder, flours, and spices and then mix together evenly. In the flour mixture, whisk in rhubarb and apple to coat.
- Whisk the milk, sugar, egg, and vanilla in another smaller bowl before pouring into the dry mixture and stirring until just combined.
- Divide the batter evenly between tins/paper cases (scatter with a few slices of rhubarb if desired) and bake for 20 minutes -25 minutes or until it rises, golden around the edges. After a skewer is inserted in the middle, it comes out cleanly.
- Remove from the oven and set aside for 5 minutes before transferring onto a wire rack to cool off further.
- Eat warm or at room temperature. It is best eaten on a baking day but will be kept for 2 days -3 days in an airtight container or frozen in zip-lock bags for longer.

Mushroom and Spinach Frittata

Prep 15 MIN
Cooking 30 MIN
Servings 4

Ingredients

- 6 eggs
- 1/4 cup (60 ml) milk
- 3 tablespoons (45 ml) butter
- 2 cups (500 ml) baby spinach
- Salt and pepper
- 1 cup grated cheddar cheese
- 1 onion, thinly sliced

- 4 oz white button mushrooms, sliced

Instructions

- Pre-heat the oven up to 180 °C (350 °F), with the rack in the middle position. Butter a baking dish of 20 cm (8") square. Set aside.
- Combine the eggs and milk in a large bowl with a whisk. Stir in cheese. Season with pepper and salt. Set aside bowl.
- Brown onion and mushrooms in butter over medium heat, in a large non-stick skillet. Season with pepper and salt. Add spinach, and continue to cook for about 1 minute, continually stirring.
- Pour the mushroom mixture into a blend of eggs. Remove well and pour over into a baking dish. Bake the frittata for about 25 mins, or until browned and puffed slightly. Cut the frittata into four squares and remove with a spatula from the platter. Place them on a plate and voila, they are ready to serve warm or cold.

Gluten-Free Crepes

Prep Time: 15 mins
Cook Time: 30 mins
Total Time: 45 mins
Servings: 10 crepes

Ingredients

Option 1. Making crepes using gluten-free and gum-free waffle and pancake mix

- 3 tablespoons sugar
- 1 1/2 cups gluten-free pancake mix
- 1 cup cold water
- 2 eggs
- 2 tablespoons butter, melted

Option 2. Making crepes using your favorite gluten-free and gum-free flour blend:

- 2 tablespoons butter, melted
- 3 tablespoons sugar
- 1 cup cold water
- 2 tablespoons cold water
- 2 eggs
- 1 1/2 cups gluten-free flour
- 1/2 tspoon gluten free baking powder or mix baking soda and cream of tartar in equal parts
- 1/2 tspoon vanilla extract

Instructions

- In a large bowl, mix all crepe ingredients, and whisk the mixture until the lumps dissolve. Allow/let the mixture sit at room temperature for some 15 minutes. After 15 minutes, it will become thickened.
- Heat the frying pan to very hot (at high heat on top of the stove), spray it with oil spray (or perhaps add melted butter) and pour a small amount of batter into the frying pan using a soup ladle or 1/4 measuring cup as you roll the pan from side-side just enough to cover the bottom of the pan evenly with a thin layer of crepe batter. You could use a whole ladle-full, or less, depending on the size of your soup ladle. That also depends on your skillet's

diameter. The trick is to cover the pan's bottom with just a slightly thick batter sheet, don't coat it too thickly.

- Depending on your pan, allow this thin layer of crepe batter to cook for 1,2 or 3 minutes (the subsequent crepes should take much less time to cook than that of the first time as the saucepan heats up more), then turn the crepe to the other side then let it cook for another minute. This way, you prepare a single crepe on each side for 1-2 minutes. To turn the crepe, catch the sides of the crepe across its circumference, slowly moving from all sides into the middle of the crepe until the crepe is removed from the pan. How to know when the time for the crepe to flip? It will get wet in the frying pan when you pour the batter, but eventually, bubbles will form, and the batter will start drying out. It's time to flip when it's all bubbles and no liquid batter!
- There's no need to spray your pan each time with a cooking spray or grease it with butter-just do it once, for the first crepe if you use a good stainless-steel pan (I use the All-Clad) or non-stick pan-spray the pan once before the first crepe is appropriate.
- The subsequent crepes that take much less time to cook, and the more you need to make, the quicker you'll need to turn the crepes because the frying pan will get heated up more and more. When you cook crepes, your frying pan is always on high heat. This will keep sticking to a minimum.
- Upon completion of each crepe, move it to the plate and place each new crepe in the stack on top of the previous crepe. Sometimes I like to brush with softened butter on each crepe and then top it with the next one (but it's not necessary). Delicious!

Amaranth Porridge with Roasted Pears

Prep Time: 10 mins
Cook Time: 30 mins
Total Time: 40 mins
Servings: 2 servings

Ingredients

- ¼ teaspoon salt
- 2 tablespoons pecan pieces
- 1 teaspoon pure maple syrup
- 1 cup plain 0% Greek yogurt, for serving
- Pears
- Porridge
- ½ cup uncooked amaranth
- 1/2 cup water
- 1 cup 2% milk
- 1 teaspoon maple syrup
- 1 large pear
- 1/2 tspoon ground cinnamon
- 1/4 tspoon ground ginger
- 1/8 tspoon ground nutmeg
- 1/8 tspoon ground clove
- Pecan/Pear Topping

Instructions

- Preheat the oven to 400 ° C.
- Drain the amaranth and rinse it. Combine with water, one cup of milk, and salt. Take the amaranth to a boil and reduce it to a simmer (all the way to low). Cover and let it cook for 25 minutes until the amaranth is soft, but

some liquid remains. Remove from heat, and allow the amaranth to thicken for another 5 to 10 minutes. If desired, apply a little more milk to smooth out the texture.

- Toss the pecan parts together with the 1 tablespoon maple syrup. Roast for 10 mins to 15 minutes, until the pecans are toasted and the maple syrup has dried. When done, pecans can become relatively fragrant. When they cool down, pecans are crisp.
- Dice the pears along with the pecans, and mix with the remaining 1 teaspoon of maple syrup and spices. Roast for 15 minutes in a roasting pan, until the pears are tender.
- In the porridge, add 3/4 of the roasted pears. Divide yogurt into two bowls and cover with porridge, pecans roasted, and the remaining bits of pear.

Turkey Apple Breakfast Hash (AIP)

Serves: about 5 portions as a breakfast

Ingredients

For the meat:

- 1 lb ground turkey
- 1 tablespoon coconut oil
- ½ teaspoon dried thyme
- ½ teaspoon cinnamon
- sea salt, to taste

For the hash:

- 1 tbspoon coconut oil
- 1 onion
- 1 large apple, peeled, cored, and chopped
- 2 cups spinach or greens of choice
- ½ tspoon turmeric
- ½ tspoon dried thyme
- sea salt, to taste
- 1 large or 2 small zucchini
- ½ cup shredded carrots
- 2 cups cubed frozen butternut squash (or the sweet potato)
- 1 tspoon cinnamon
- ¾ tspoon powdered ginger
- ½ tspoon garlic powder

Instructions

- In a skillet heat a spoonful of coconut oil over medium/high heat. Attach turkey to the ground and cook until crispy. Season with thyme, cinnamon, and a pinch of sea salt. Moving to plate.
- Throw remaining coconut oil into the same skillet and sauté onion until softened for 2-3 minutes.
- Add the courgettes, apple, carrots, and frozen squash to taste—Cook for around 4-5 minutes, or until veggies soften.
- Attach and whisk in spinach until wilted.
- Add cooked turkey, seasoning, salt, and shut off oil.
- Enjoy this hash fresh from the pan, or let it cool and refrigerate all week long. The hash can remain in a sealed container in the refrigerator for about 5-6 days.

No-Bake Chocolate Chia Energy Bars

Prep Time: 10 mins
Total Time: 10 mins
Servings: 14 bars

Ingredients

- 1 ½ cups packed, pitted dates
- 1/2 cup unsweetened shredded coconut
- 1 cup raw walnut pieces
- 1/4 cup (35 g) raw cocoa powder or cocoa powder
- 1/2 cup (75 g) whole chia seeds
- 1/2 cup (70 g) chopped dark chocolate
- 1/2 cup (50 g) oats
- 1 teasp pure vanilla extract, optional, enhances the flavour
- 1/4 teasp unrefined sea salt, optional, enhances the flavour

Instructions

- Place the dates in a blender or food processor and purée until thick paste forms are formed.
- Add the walnuts and blend to mix.
- Add the remaining ingredients and combine until a thick dough is formed.
- Line a rectangular parchment-papered baking pan. Place the mixture tightly in the pan and place straight into all corners.
- Place in the freezer until midnight, for at least a few hours.
- Raise from the pan and cut into 14 strips.

- Place in the refrigerator or an airtight container.

Nutrition Info

Serving Size: 1 bar Sugar: 17 g Fat: 12 g Calories: 234 calories
Carbohydrates: 28 g Protein: 4.5 g Fiber: 7 g

Buckwheat Cinnamon and Ginger Granola

Servings: 4

Ingredients:

- ¼ cup Chia seeds
- ½ Cup Coconut Flakes
- 1 ½ Cup mixed Raw nuts – I love almonds, pecans, hazelnuts and walnuts
- 2 cups of gluten-free oats
- 1 cup of buckwheat groats
- 2 tbsp nut butter
- 4 tbsp of coconut oil
- 1 cup of sunflower seeds
- ½ cup of pumpkin seeds
- 1 ½ - 2 inches piece of ginger
- 1 tsp Ground Cinnamon
- 1/3 cup of Rice Malt Syrup or Raw Honey
- 4 tbsp of raw cacao powder – Optional

Instructions:

- Preheat the oven up to 180C
- Put the nuts in your food processor and quickly blitz to chop roughly. Place the chopped nuts in a large mixing

bowl and add all the other dry ingredients that combine well–oats, coconut, cinnamon, buckwheat, seeds, and salt In a low heat saucepan, melt the coconut oil gently,

- Add the cacao powder (if used) to the wet mixture and blend well Pour the wet mixture over the dry mixture then mix well to make sure that everything is coated Move the mixture to a wide baking tray lined with grease-proof paper or coconut oil greased. Be sure to uniformly distribute the mixture for 35-40 minutes, turning the mixture halfway through. Bake until the granola is fresh and golden!
- Allow the granola to cool and store in an airtight container for up to 2 weeks before putting it in.
- Serve with your favorite nut milk, coconut yogurt scoop, fresh fruit and superfoods–goji berries, flax seeds, bee pollen, whatever you like! Mix it up every single day.

Foolproof Spinach and Feta Frittata

Servings 4

Ingredients

- 1 tsp olive oil
- ½ small brown onion peeled and finely sliced
- 1 tsp garlic
- 250 g baby spinach
- 4 eggs
- ½ cup crumbled feta cheese
- Salt and pepper to taste

Instructions

- Pre-heat the grill to medium-high heat.
- Heat the oil over medium heat using a non-stick frying pan, which you can place under the grill.
- Add the onion and cook until just brown. Remove the spinach and toss for one or two minutes, until it starts to wilt. Remove from heat and allow to refrigerate.
- In a bowl, crack the eggs. Attach the spinach and onion, then the feta, cooled in—taste season.
- Put the frying saucepan back on medium heat and add the eggs. Stir gently with a spatula until you notice that the egg starts to set at the bottom. Switch off the heat, so that the frittata stays runny.
- Put your frying pan under the grill for 2 minutes to 3 minutes, or until the frittata is golden and cooked all the

way through (check with a fork). Place/put a plate over the saucepan and turn over quickly but carefully to release frittata. Serve in a crispy side salad, hot or cold.

Nutrition Info

Calories: 153

Quick and Easy Quinoa Orange Salad

Serving 1

Ingredients

- 20g Brazil nuts, chopped
- 1 green onion, sliced
- 1 cup cooked quinoa, cooled
- 2 small oranges, supremed
- 1 celery rib, finely chopped
- ¼ cup fresh parsley, finely chopped

For the dressing

- juice from above oranges
- ½ tsp lemon juice
- ½ tsp salt
- ¼ tsp black pepper
- pinch cinnamon
- ½ tsp fresh ginger, grated
- 1 tsp white wine vinegar
- 1 small clove garlic, minced

- Cut the oranges into supremes, operate over a bowl, so that none of the juice is lost. When all of the supremes are finished, make sure to suck all of the juice out of the "membranes" left behind.
- Move the juice to your food processor or mini blender. Add the remaining ingredients to the dressing, then blend until smooth.
- Cut your supreme orange into bits of bite-size, and add them to a mixing bowl of medium size. Attach remaining ingredients, like sauce, and stir well until combined.
- Eat right away, or hold in the fridge until ready to serve.

Lettuce Wraps with Smoked Trout

4 servings

Ingredients

- 2 medium carrots, peeled
- 1/2 unpeeled English hothouse cucumber (don't remove seeds)
- 1 tbspoon sugar
- 1 tbspoon fish sauce (such as nam pla or nuoc nam)
- 2 4.5-oz packages skinless smoked trout fillets, broken into bite-size pieces (about 2 cups)
- 1/3 cup Asian sweet chili sauce
- 1/4 cup dry-roasted peanuts (finely chopped lightly salted)
- 1/4 cup thinly sliced shallots
- 1/4 cup thinly sliced jalapeño chiles with seeds
- 2 tbspoons fresh lime juice or unseasoned rice vinegar

- 1 cup diced grape tomatoes
- 16 small to medium inner leaves of romaine lettuce (from about 2 hearts of romaine)
- 1/2 cup whole fresh mint leaves
- 1/2 cup small whole fresh basil leaves

Instructions

- Shave carrots and cucumber lengthwise into ribbons using a vegetable peeler. Cut the ribbons into three-inch-long sections, then cut sections into strips of match size—place in a big bowl. Stir in shallots, jalapeños, lime juice, sugar, and fish sauce; let marinate at room temperature for 30 minutes.
- Add bits of trout and tomatoes to the vegetable mixture, then toss to match. Switch mixture of trout to a large strainer and rinse off liquid. Return the mix of trout and vegetables to the same bowl; add mint and basil, and swirl to blend.
- Arrange leaves of lettuce on a large platter. Divide the lettuce leaves into lettuce salads. Drizzle each salad with sweet chili sauce and sprinkle with peanuts.

Nutrition Info

Calories 423
Carbohydrates 60 g (20%)
Fat 12 g (18%)
Protein33 g (65%)
Saturated Fat 2 g (9%)
Sodium 1245 mg (52%)

Winter Fruit Salad with, Pears, Grapes, Persimmons, and Pecans

Serving: 6 side-dish servings

Total Time: 25 minutes
Prep Time: 25 minutes

Ingredients:

- 3/4 cup pecans, cut into 1/2 lengthwise to make slivers
- 4 Fuyu persimmons, cut in 1 inch cubes
- 3 Bosch pears, cut in 1 inch cubes
- 1 cup grapes, cut into 2 or 4 if large

Dressing Ingredients:

- 1 T peanut oil
- 1 T pomegranate-flavored vinegar
- 2 T agave nectar or any sweetener of your choice
- 1 T extra virgin olive oil
- pinch of salt, to taste

Instructions:

- Whisk the dressing ingredients together so that the flavors will mix while the fruit is being cut. Sliced the grapes, the persimmons, and the pears into bits of the same size (about 1 inch) and put them in a plastic bowl. Toss the fruit and dress it up. Shortly before serving, throw on pieces of pecan.

Other fruits like figs, apples, or pomegranate arils could be used to replace any of these, but you need 5 cups -6 cups of cut fruit.

Roasted Red Pepper and Sweet Potato Soup

Prep Time: 25 minutes
Cook Time: 30 minutes
Total Time: 55 minutes
6 servings

Ingredients

- 1 can (4 oz) diced green chiles
- 2 teaspoons ground cumin
- 4 cups vegetable broth
- 2 tablespoons minced fresh cilantro
- 1 tablespoon lemon juice
- 4 oz cream cheese, cubed
- 2 tbspoons olive oil
- 2 medium onions, chopped
- 1 jar (12 ounces) roasted red peppers, chopped, liquid reserved
- 1 tspoon salt
- 1 tspoon ground coriander
- 3 – 4 cups cubed sweet potatoes (peeled)

Instructions

- Heat the olive oil over medium-high heat in a big soup pot or Dutch oven. Adding the onion and cook until soft.

Add red peppers, green chiles, cumin, salt, and cilantro to taste—Cook for about 1-2 minutes.

- Add roasted red peppers, sweet potatoes, and vegetable broth to the reserved juice. Bring to a boil and reduce heat, then cover.
- Cook for 10-15 minutes, until the potatoes are tender. Stir in the juice of the cilantro and lemon. Let the soup cool off a little bit.
- Place half of the soup and the cream cheese into a blender. Process until smooth, then put in the soup pot again and heat through. Season with extra salt, if necessary.

Smoked Salmon Potato Tartine

Prep Time: 25 minutes
Cook Time: 20 minutes
Total Time: 45 minutes
2 Servings

Ingredients

Potato Tartine:

- 1 big russet potato, peeled and grated lengthwise
- salt
- pepper
- 2 tbspoons clarified butter (or other neutral-flavored oil)

Toppings:

- 1/2 garlic clove, finely minced
- zest of half a lemon

- 4 oz soft goat cheese
- 1 1/2 tbspoons finely minced chives
- thinly sliced smoked salmon
- 2 tablespoons drained capers
- finely minced chives (for garnish)
- 2 tablespoons finely chopped red onion
- 1/2 hard-boiled egg, finely chopped

Instructions:

Assemble Toppings:

- In a small bowl, add lemon zest, goat's cheese, and garlic. Season to taste, use salt and pepper. Stir gently in fresh chives. Set aside.
- Spice the sliced red onion with salt and hard-boiled egg.

Preparation of Potato Tartine:

- Working quickly (as the potato would start oxidizing quickly), grate the potato (longitudinally) into a wide using a grater's large holes. To remove any excess liquid, squeeze the potatoes over the sink. Season with salt and pepper, and shake generously.
- Heat clarified butter over medium to high heat in an 8-10 inch non-stick skillet. When dry, add the grated potato to a large circle and shape it roughly, using a spatula.
- To compact, cover and cook gently for 8-10 minutes or until the bottom is golden brown, press that mixture with the back of the spoon.
- Flip to the other side carefully and cook for another 8-10 minutes, or until golden brown and crispy.

- Take from the rack to cool and allow to cool until the temperature is barely lukewarm or roomy.

Assemble Tartine:

- Once the potato cake has cooled, spread the mixture of the goat cheese over the edges. Cover directly over the smoked salmon and scatter with the red onion, hard-boiled egg, and capers. Garnish with chives, freshly sliced.
- Cut into wedges, and instantly serve.

Buddha Bowl with Orange, Avocado, Kale, and Wild Rice

Prep: 10 min
Cook: 30 min
Total: 40 min
2 servings

Ingredients

Rice

- 1 cup wild rice
- 3 cups vegetable broth or water
- 1 garlic clove, minced
- 2 tablespoons extra-virgin olive oil
- 2 tablespoons rice vinegar
- 1 tablespoon chopped fresh mint
- Salt and freshly ground black pepper

Toppings

- 1 bunch kale, roughly chopped
- 2 tablespoons olive oil
- 1 tablespoon rice vinegar
- ¼ cup pomegranate seeds
- 1 orange, cut into segments
- ½ avocado, sliced
- ¼ cup pumpkin seeds
- 2 hard-boiled eggs
- Salt and freshly ground black pepper

Instructions

- Make the Rice: Mix the rice with the broth (or tea, if used) and garlic in a medium pot to mix. Bring in the mixture over medium-high heat to a simmer.

- When the liquid is boiling, reduce heat to low and simmer for 15 to 17 minutes until the rice is tender and all the liquid is absorbed.

- Let the rice cool for 5 to 10 minutes, then add the olive oil, vinegar, mint, salt, and pepper to stir.

- Make the Toppings: Throw the kale with the olive oil and the vinegar in a medium bowl. Divide the rice into two bowls, then cover with fair kale.

- Cover each of the bowls with 2 tablespoons of pomegranate seeds, half of the orange slices, half the slices of avocado, 2 tablespoons of pumpkin seeds, and one hard-boiled egg. Season with salt and pepper over the egg. Serve straight away.

Nutrition Info

Rice

417 calories
15g fat
62g carbs
12g protein
2g sugars

Toppings

453 calories
34g fat
28g carbs
16g protein

Beetroot, Lentil, and Hazelnut Salad With a Ginger Dressing

Active Time 10 minutes
Total Time 10 minutes
Serves 2–3

Ingredients

For the salad:

- Sea salt

- 3 cooked beetroot, cut into small cubes
- A handful of fresh mint, roughly chopped
- 2 spring onions, finely sliced
- A handful of fresh parsley, roughly chopped
- 1 cup Puy lentils, rinsed
- 2 3/4 cup filtered water
- 2 tbpoons hazelnuts, roughly chopped

For the ginger dressing:

- 3/4-inch cube of fresh ginger, peeled and roughly chopped
- 1 tablespoon apple cider vinegar
- Pinch of sea salt and ground black pepper (freshly)
- 6 tablepoons olive oil
- 1 teaspoon Dijon mustard

Instructions

- Put them in a casserole for the lentils, cover with water, bring the heat to a boil, and simmer for around 15–20 minutes or until all the liquid has evaporated and the lentils are not mushy and still have a bite.
- Once the lentils have been cooked, move them into a large bowl and leave to cool.
- Add the beetroot, hazelnuts, spring onions, and herbs once the lentils are cold, and mix until all is combined.
- Place the ginger, mustard, oil, and vinegar in a bowl for the dressing and mix until mixed using a hand-held blender.
- Drizzle the salad over its dressing and serve.

Nutrition Info

Calories815
Carbohydrates78 g (26%)
Fat46 g (71%)
Protein28 g (55%)
Saturated Fat6 g (31%)
Sodium1486 mg (62%)

Herb-Crusted Cauliflower Steaks with Beans and Tomatoes

Active Time 30 minutes
Total Time 45 minutes
2 servings

Ingredients

- 2 teaspoons kosher salt, divided
- 1 teaspoon freshly ground black pepper, divided
- 8 ounces green beans, trimmed
- 1 (15-oz) can white beans, rinsed, drained
- 1 cp golden or red cherry tomatoes (about 6 oz), halved
- 1/3 cup panko (Japanese breadcrumbs)
- 1/4 cup freshly grated Parmesan
- 3 tbspoons mayonnaise
- 1 tspoon Dijon mustard
- 1 large head of cauliflower (around 2 pounds)
- 1/2 cp olive oil, divided
- 3 garlic cloves, finely chopped
- 3/4 tspoon finely grated lemon zest
- 1/3 cp chopped parsley, plus more for serving

- Arrange a middle and upper third of oven racks; pre-heat to 425 ° F. Remove the leaves and cut the cauliflower end of the stem, and leave the heart intact. Place the center of the cauliflower down on a surface of work. Slice in the middle from top to bottom, using a large knife, to produce 2 (1)" "steaks; "save the remaining cauliflower for another use.
- Place the cauliflower on a baking sheet that is rimmed. Brush with 1 Tbsp on both sides. Oil; 1/4 tsp for the season. Salt, 1/4 tsp. Pepper, pepper. Roast on the middle rack, rotating for about 30 minutes until the cauliflower is tender and brown.
- Then toss 1 Tbsp of green beans. Carbon, 1/2 dc. Salt, with 1/4 tsp. Pepper over another sheet of rimmed baking. Set aside in a single layer, then roast in the upper third of the oven until green beans start blistering, around 15 min.
- Whisk on garlic, lemon zest, 1/3 cup parsley, and 6 Tbsp remaining. Oil, with 1 1/4 tsp. Salt, 1/2 tablespoon. Pepper until smooth, in a medium bowl. Pass half the blend to another medium bowl. Attach panko and parmesan to the bowl first, then combine with hands. In the second bowl, add white beans and tomatoes, and toss to coat. In a small bowl, mix mayonnaise and mustard.
- Remove sheets from the frying pan. Spread the mixture of mayonnaise over the cauliflower. Sprinkle the mixture with 1/4 cup panko uniformly over the cauliflower. Add white bean mixture with green beans to the board, and toss to blend. Put back the sheets to the oven and continue to roast until the white beans start to crisp, and

the panko topping starts to brown for another 5–7 minutes.

- Divide into plates, the cauliflower, white beans, green beans, and tomatoes. Top with some parsley.

Note.

Cut one big part from a cauliflower head, keeping the center root intact. Use 2 large cauliflower heads to serve 4. Roast remaining cauliflower alongside" steaks "or integrate them into soup, salad, or other use. Substitute in vegan mayonnaise for standard mayonnaise for a vegan version.

Nutrition Info

Calories1141
Fat77 g (119%)
Polyunsaturated Fat17 g
Fiber25 g (98%)
Carbohydrates89 g (30%)
Protein34 g (68%)
Saturated Fat13 g (66%)
Sodium2287 mg (95%)
Monounsaturated Fat45 g
Cholesterol18 mg (6%)

Grilled Sauerkraut Avocado Sandwich

Tangy sauerkraut, crunchy with creamy avocado and hummus stuffed in between two slices of pumpernickel bread and grilled until soft and crispy!

Prep Time 10 minutes

Cook Time 12 minutes
Total Time 22 minutes
Servings 4

Ingredients

- 1 cup hummus (roasted garlic flavor, divided)
- 1 cup sauerkraut (drained, lightly rinsed, and liquid squeezed out)
- 8 slices pumpernickel bread
- vegan buttery spread (or regular butter)
- 1 avocado (peeled and sliced lengthwise into about 16 pieces (If you want to lower the fat content of the sandwich, you can leave this ingredient out, and it will still be very delicious!))

Instructions

- Pre-heat the oven up to 450 degrees F (230 degrees C).
- Spread the butter on one side of each of the eight slices of bread, and put 4 of them butter side down on a baking sheet.
- Take approximately half the hummus and spread over 4 slices of bread.
- Distribute a single slice of the sauerkraut over the hummus.
- Distribute slices of avocado over the sauerkraut.
- Place hummus on the side without butter for the remaining 4 slices of bread and put hummus side down onto the avocado slices.
- Bake for 6-8 minutes in the oven, then turn the sandwiches and bake for another 6 mins, until the sandwiches are golden brown and crispy. (Alternatively,

you can barbecue them on a griddle or skillet on the top of the stove).

Nutrition Info

Calories 319
Calories from Fat 126
Total Fat 14g 22%
Saturated Fat 2g 10%
Sodium 781mg

Glowing Spiced Lentil Soup

Prep time 15 Minutes
Cook time 20 Minutes
7 cups (1.65 liters)

Ingredients:

- 1/4 tspoon ground cardamom
- 1 (15-oz/398 mL) can diced tomatoes, with juices
- 1 (15-oz/398 mL) can full-fat coconut milk*
- 1 1/2 tbspoons extra-virgin olive oil
- 2 cups diced onion (1 medium/large)
- 2 large garlic cloves, minced
- Freshly ground black pepper, to taste
- Red pepper flakes/cayenne pepper, to taste (for a kick of heat!)
- 1 (5-oz/140-gram) package baby spinach
- 2 tspoons fresh lime juice, or more to taste
- 2 tspoons ground turmeric
- 1 1/2 teaspoons ground cumin
- 1/2 teaspoon cinnamon
- 3/4 cp uncooked red lentils, rinsed and drained
- 3 1/2 cps (875 mL) low-sodium vegetable broth
- 1/2 tspoon fine sea salt, or to taste

Instructions:

- Place the onion, oil, and garlic in a large saucepan. Add a pinch of salt, mix and sauté for 4 to 5 minutes over medium heat until the onion has softened.
- To combine, add the turmeric, cinnamon, cumin, and cardamom. Continue cooking, until fragrant, for about 1 minute.
- Attach the diced tomatoes (with juice), whole coconut milk can, red lentils, broth, salt, and lots of pepper. Where desired, add red pepper flakes or cayenne to taste. Stir to combine. Increase to high heat and carry to a low boil.
- Reduce heat to medium-high once it boils and simmer, uncovered, for about 18 to 22 minutes until the lentils are fluffy and tender.
- Turn off the heat until wilted and whisk in the spinach. Stir in the lime juice to taste. If needed, sauté and add more salt and pepper. Ladle into bowls and serve with toasted lime wedges and bread.

Kale Pesto Bulgur Salad Recipe

Serves 4-6

Ingredients

- 1/2 (half) pound green beans, trimmed and cut into bite-sized pieces
- 1/4 cup plus 3 Tbsp. sliced almonds, toasted, plus more for garnish
- 1 garlic clove
- 1 cup stemmed and thinly sliced lacinato kale (from about 1/2 bunch)

- 1/2 cup packed basil leaves
- 1/4 cup extra-virgin olive oil
- 1/4 cup lemon juice (starting from about 2 lemons)
- 1/2 tsp. kosher salt
- 1 1/2 cups bulgur
- 1 tsp. kosher salt, divided, plus more to taste
- 1 pint grape tomatoes, halved
- 1/4 packed flat-leaf parsley
- 3 Tbsp. sliced almonds
- 1/4 tsp. ground black pepper

Instructions

To make the salad:

- Soak bulgur and 1/2 tsp in a large bowl. Heat overnight in 3 cups of water. If necessary, drain. (Alternatively, bring 3 cups of water to a boil, then pour over bulgur into a heat-proof bowl, cover, and let sit for 25 minutes. Drain and allow to cool to room temperature.)

- Pulse garlic until chopped in a food processor equipped with a metal blade. Add kale, basil, parsley, and 1/4 tablespoon almonds and pulse until finely chopped. Apply the oil, the lemon juice, and 1/2 tsp remaining. Season with salt and pepper, and puree until soft.

- Move pesto to a bulgur dish. Add the green beans, tomatoes, and remaining 3 Tbsp. Combine almonds and toss well. Garnish and serve with extra almonds.

Curried Red Lentil and Swiss Chard Soup

Servings: Serves 6

Ingredients

- 2 tablespoons olive oil
- 1 large onion, thinly sliced
- pound (1 bunch) Swiss chard, tough stalks removed, coarsely chopped
- 2 cups (about 14 oz) dried red lentils
- 5 tspoons curry powder
- 1 tspoon salt
- 6 tbspoons thick Greek yogurt, thinned with 2 tbspoons water
- 1 red/green jalapeño chili, stemmed and thinly sliced
- 1 lime, cut into 6 wedges
- 1/4 teaspoon ground red pepper (cayenne)
- 5 cups vegetable broth
- 1 can (15-ounce) chickpeas, rinsed and drained

Instructions

- Heat the oil over medium heat in a large, heavy saucepan. Attach onion; cook for about 10 minutes, frequently stirring, until lightly golden. Stir in red pepper and curry. Add 4 cups of broth and chard; heat up and bring to a boil, stirring until the chard wilts.

- Stir in chickpeas and lentils. Reduce the heat to low, cover then simmer for 16 to 18 minutes until lentils are tender, stirring twice.

- Take off heat. Puree half the soup in a blender/food processor (about 4 cups); return the purée to the bowl. Adding the remaining 1 cup of broth and salt, and steam for 2 minutes over low heat.

- Divide the soup into 6 bowls. Drizzle the thinned yogurt about 1 tablespoon over each serving—garnish with some jalapeño slices and a lime wedge.

Smoked salmon salad with green goddess dressing

0:15 Prep
0:20 Cook
4 Servings Easy

Ingredients

- 1/2 cup French green lentils, rinsed
- 2 baby fennel bulbs, some fronds reserved (thinly sliced)
- 130g (1/2 cup) natural yogurt
- 2 tbspoons chopped fresh continental parsley, plus extra parsley leaves, to serve
- Pinch of caster sugar
- 60g baby spinach
- 1/2 avocado, sliced
- 180g sliced salt-reduced smoked salmon
- 2 tbspoons chopped fresh chives
- 1 tbspoon chopped fresh tarragon
- 1 tbspoon salted baby capers, rinsed, drained
- 1 tspoon finely grated lemon rind
- 1/2 red onion, thinly sliced

- 1 tbspoon fresh lemon juice

Instructions

- Cook lentils for 20 mins or until tender, in a large saucepan of boiling water. Drain and drain.
- In the meantime, heat a pan of chargrilling over high heat. Spray oil on slices of fennel. Cook each side for 2 mins, or until tender.
- In a food processor, process the yogurt, tarragon, capers, parsley, chives, and lemon rind until smooth—season with potatoes.
- In a bowl, place the sugar, onion, juice, and a pinch of salt. Place some 5 minutes aside. Drain and drain.
- In a large bowl, mix the lentils, onion, spinach, fennel, and avocado. Divide between plates—top on salmon. Sprinkle with the fronds of the reserved fennel and extra parsley. Drizzle with dressing green goddess.

Miso Soup

2 servings

Ingredients

For dashi (or substitute 2 cups water, chicken broth, or vegetable broth):

- 2 cups of water
- 1 (2inch) piece kombu (dried black kelp)
- 1/2 cup loosely packed dried bonito flakes (katsuobushi), optional

For the miso soup:

- 4 ounces silken or firm tofu, drained
- 1 to 2 medium scallions
- 2 tablespoons red or white miso paste

Instructions

- Make dashi; Combine the water and the kombu over medium heat in a 1 quarter saucepan. Take off the kombu just as the water begins to boil. If using, apply the bonito flakes and let the water cool down quickly. Simmer for about 1 minute, then heat off the pan and let the bonito steep for another 5 minutes. Strain out the dashi bonito. Add additional water to make 2 cups, if necessary. Conversely, substitute 2 cup water, chicken broth, or vegetable broth.

- Have tofu and scallions prepared. Break the tofu into tiny cubes on each side, 1/4-inch to 1/2-inch. Pick rather thinly on the scallions.

- Take the broth to a fast simmer. Add the dashi or broth back into the saucepan, and over medium-high heat carry to a rapid simmer.

- Mix the miso and 1/2 cup hot broth together. Place the miso in a tiny ramekin or measure cup. Scoop the broth out about 1/2 cup and spill over the miso. Mix with a fork/whisk until the miso dissolves completely in the water, and no lumps are remaining.

- Load the miso into the frying pan. Place the dissolved miso into the broth to cook.

- Stir in tofu. Lower the heat to medium-low and add the miso tofu. Simmer for 1 to 2 minutes, just enough to cook the tofu. Do not boil the miso once you have removed the tofu.

- Attach some scallions. Scatter the scallions on the top of the broth just before serving.

- Serving in small bowls. Pour the miso into bowls, then serve. Miso is best served when fresh. As it remains in the water, it will calm down a bit; whisk quickly with chopsticks or a spoon to mix/stir the soup again.

Nutrition Info

Calories 123
Fat 6 g (9.3%)
Saturated 0.9 g (4.7%)
Carbs 8.5 g (2.8%)
Fiber 2.6 g (10.4%)
Sugars 1.4 g
Protein

Healing Carrot Soup with Turmeric and Ginger

Prep 5 mins
Cook 15 mins
Total 20 mins

Servings 2

Ingredients

- 3 cups low sodium vegetable broth, warm
- 1 tspoon turmeric powder
- 1-inch ginger knob, peeled and grated
- Juice from 1/2 of a lemon
- Pinch cayenne pepper
- 4 carrots, peeled and chopped
- 1 parsnip, peeled and chopped
- 1 yellow onion, roughly chopped
- 4 garlic cloves, crushed
- 2 tspoons virgin coconut oil
- Fresh parsley, black sesame, Greek yogurt, coconut flakes, to serve

Instructions

- Pre-heat the oven to 350oF.
- Top a parchment-papered baking sheet. Attach the onion, carrots, parsnip, and garlic, then season with turmeric and cayenne, drizzle with coconut oil and mix evenly to cover.
- Remove from the oven and switch to a mixer with vegetable broth, lemon juice, and ginger for 15 minutes.
- Blend the ingredients until creamy and smooth.
- Pour the soup into serving cups, garnish with fresh parsley, flakes of sesame and coconut, cut with Greek yogurt, and serve warmly.

Lemony Lentil Soup

Prep Time 5 minutes
Cook Time 1 hour 30 minutes
Total Time 1 hour 35 minutes

Ingredients

- 2 1/2 (32 ounces) boxes vegetable broth
- 2 tspoons dried turmeric
- 1 1/2 cps diced or sliced carrots
- 1 1/2 cps diced celery (1 full head)
- 1 tspoon salt
- 3 cloves garlic, minced
- 1 tablespoon extra virgin olive oil
- 1 yellow onion, diced
- 4 teaspoons fresh grated ginger
- 2 cps green lentils, rinsed and picked over for stones
- zest of 1/2 lemon
- juice of 3 small lemons

Instructions

- Heat oil on medium heat in a big Dutch oven. Add the celery, onion, carrots, salt and sauté for about 5 minutes until softened. Add an additional minute of garlic and ginger and sauté. Stir in the broth, turmeric, and lentils.
- Reduce heat to low and then simmer for 45 minutes, partially covered. Attach the zest of lemon and juice and cook for another 30 minutes. If needed, add more broth.

Nutrition Info

Calories: 122
Total Fat: 2g
Saturated Fat: 0g

Greek Salad Chicken Wrap

Prep time 10 mins
Cook time 35 mins
Total time 45 mins
Serves: 2

Ingredients

For the chicken:

- 2 bone-in chicken breasts
- 1 tbspoon olive oil

small shakes of the following per chicken breast:

- lemon pepper
- dried oregano
- garlic powder

For the Greek salad:

- 4 cups romaine, chopped
- fresh lemon wedges (optional)
- whole wheat or gluten-free wraps
- 2 tablespoons hummus per wrap
- ½ cup cucumber slices, sliced, then halved

- 2 tablespoons kalamata olives
- ¼ cup feta cheese
- red wine vinegar
- ¼ cup cherry tomatoes, sliced
- ¼ cup red onion
- olive oil

Instructions

- To make chicken: Pre-heat oven to 375 degrees for the chicken. Line a foil baking sheet with 1/2 tablespoon of oil and drizzle. Put 2 chicken breasts bone-in on top and season with salt, pepper, dried oregano, and lemon pepper. Add 1/2 tbspoon of olive oil and bake for 35-40 minutes or until chicken is cooked. With this cover using immediately or as leftovers. There is going to be enough chicken for four big wraps.
- Making the salad: Place the chopped romaine in a bowl. Finish with cherry tomatoes, red onion, cucumbers, feta cheese, and olives. Sprinkle with some dried orégano shakes. Use the vinegar to dress, and go around the bowl for two turns. With the olive oil, go around once. Squeeze fresh lemon juice (1 big wedge is fine) over everything. If required, stir and adjust seasonings.
- To make wrap: spread 2 tablespoons of hummus over your chosen wrap. A heaping piece of Greek salad, top with slices of chicken. Rolling, wrapping, and devouring!

Shrimp Bok Choy and Turmeric Soup

Prep Time: 20 mins
Cook Time: 30 mins
Total Time: 50 mins
Servings: 4

Ingredients

- 1 1/2 tspoon Salt, plus additional for serving
- 1 pound Shitake Mushrooms, stems removed and sliced into 1/2 inch pieces
- 1 tspoon Ground Black Pepper, plus additional for serving (optional for AIP)
- 1 tspoon Turmeric
- 1 tablespoon Extra Virgin Olive Oil
- 1 large Onion, chopped
- 6 (bottoms chopped off) heads Baby Bok Choy
- 6 Garlic Cloves, minced
- 1 pound Shrimp
- 6 cups Chicken Broth
- 2 Carrots, sliced

Instructions

- Heat the oil in a stockpot/dutch oven over medium heat.
- Add garlic and onions and then sauté for 5 minutes or until translucent.
- Add salt, pepper, turmeric, chicken broth, carrots, and mushrooms and bring to a boil. Reduce heat and cook for 20 minutes, covered.
- In the last 5 mins of cooking, add the bok choy and shrimp.
- Season with salt and pepper and drink.

Kale, Chickpea and Tomato Stew Recipe

Active time: 30 minutes
Total time: 40 minutes
Serves 4

Ingredients

- 4 Tbsp. olive oil, divided
- 4 large eggs
- 6 garlic cloves, thinly sliced
- 1/4 tsp. crushed red pepper flakes
- 1 medium onion, cut into eighths
- 1 1/4 tsp. kosher salt, divided
- 2 (15-ounce) cans chickpeas, drained and rinsed
- 1 cup vegetable stock
- 3/4 pound kale, stems removed and leaves coarsely chopped
- 1 pound tomatoes (around 3 medium), cored and chopped

Instructions

- Heat up 2 Tbsp in a large saucepan oil over low to medium heat. Add 1/4 tsp of onion. Salt and cook for about 7 minutes until tender. Add the garlic and red pepper flakes and cook for another 2 minutes. Attach the kale and stir for about 2 minutes, until wilted. Add chickpeas, tomatoes, and stock; cook over medium heat until tomatoes begin breaking down, around 10 minutes. Season on 3/4 tsp. Salt.

- Heat remaining 2 Tbsp in a big non-stick skillet. Oil over moderate heat. Crack in 2 eggs and cook for about 3 minutes, until lightly crisp on the bottom and whites. Switch to a pan, and repeat with 2 eggs leftover. Spoon stew into 4 shallow bowls, each with a fried egg on top, sprinkle with 1/4 tsp remaining. Season with salt and drink.

Turmeric Chickpea Cakes

Serves 4
Prep and Cook time: 15 minutes

Ingredients

- 1 small onion
- 2 tablespoons potato starch
- 1-2 teaspoons of sea salt
- 2 cloves of garlic
- 1/2 – 1 tspoon cayenne pepper (optional)
- 2 tbspoons chickpea flour + extra 3 tablespoons for coating
- grapeseed oil for cooking
- 1 can rinsed and drained chickpeas
- freshly ground black pepper
- 1 tspoon turmeric powder

Instructions:

- Drizzle a little grapeseed oil in a large cast-iron pan and fry the onion and garlic until it is slightly golden but not burnt. Take off heat and allow to cool.

- In the food processor, put the chickpeas until they turn to a finely textured paste, make sure to turn off your food processor, and then scrape down the sides to grind up all the chickpeas. Add the onion and garlic, salt, vinegar, pepper, turmeric, and cayenne pepper and blend well.

Switch off the food processor, whisk in the chopped parsley.

- (If you have children, you could skip the cayenne pepper altogether as most children aren't in spicy foods. Or split the batch into two and season them differently for kids and adults.) Take a large plate and sprinkle with some tbspoons of chickpea flour. Scoop some mixture with a spoon on your hands and shape it into a sphere, the size of a golf ball, and gently press to make a patty. Fall into the chickpea flour for even coating. If too much flour stays on the patty, then dust it gently with your fingertips or a pastry brush. All the patties/burgers should have a very light coating.

- Heat that same large iron cast pan to medium heat. Drizzle with a little bit more oil and put the patties into a cook. Cook on each side for about 2-3 minutes, until well browned at the bottom.

- For a balanced lunch or dinner, serve with a large salad. Or for kids with cutting vegetables to the side. Makes a great party tablecloth or party dish of potluck! Love it!

Turmeric Roasted Chickpeas

Prep Time:10 minutes
Cook Time:40 minutes
Total Time:50 minutes
Servings:15 ounces

Ingredients

- 1 teaspoon turmeric
- 1/2 teaspoon paprika
- 1/4 teaspoon black pepper
- 1 teaspoon salt
- 2 teaspoon olive or grapeseed oil
- 1 can chickpeas (garbanzo beans)

Instructions

- Open the can of chickpeas and rinse.
- Toss the chickpeas with salt, olive oil, and spices on a lined baking sheet (parchment, Silpat, or tinfoil will do).
- Bake for another 20 minutes. Jiggle the pan to push the chickpeas around, and make sure they still cook. Bake 20 more minutes, then remove to cool.
- Keep in a jar or plastic bag at room temperature if you don't eat them all right away...

- SpoonTip: Taste one raw and change the flavors to suit your needs.

Roasted Salmon with Smoky Chickpeas and Greens

Prep 40 m
Total Time: 40 m
4 servings

Ingredients

- ¼ teaspoon garlic powder
- 10 cups chopped kale
- 1 (15 ounces) can no-salt-added chickpeas, rinsed
- 1/4 cup buttermilk
- ¼ cup mayonnaise
- 1¼ pounds wild salmon, cut into 4 portions
- 2 tablespoons extra-virgin olive oil, divided
- 1 tbspoon smoked paprika
- ½ tspoon salt, divided, plus a pinch
- ¼ cp chopped fresh chives and/or dill, plus more for garnish
- ½ tspoon ground pepper, divided
- ¼ cup of water

Instructions

- In the upper third and middle of the oven, put racks; pre-heat to 425 ° F. In a medium bowl, mix 1 spoonful of butter, paprika and 1/4 teaspoon of salt. Pat chickpeas dry very thoroughly, then toss with the paprika mixture.

- Spread over a baking sheet, rimmed. Bake the chickpeas on top rack for 30 minutes, stirring frequently. Alternatively, in a blender, until creamy, puree buttermilk, mayonnaise, spices, 1/4 teaspoon pepper, and garlic powder.
- Set aside. Heat up the remaining 1 tbspoon of oil over medium heat in a large skillet. Add the kale, and cook for 2 minutes, stirring occasionally.
- Add water and continue cooking, about 5 minutes longer, until the kale is tender. Remove from heat, and add salt in a pinch.
- From the oven, remove the chickpeas and transfer them to one side of the pan. Place the salmon on the other hand, and season each salt and pepper with the remaining 1/4 teaspoon. Bake for 5 minutes to 8 minutes, until the salmon is just cooked.
- Drizzle the reserved salmon dressing, garnish with more herbs if desired, and serve with the chickpeas and kale.

Nutrition Info

447 calories; 23 g carbohydrates22 g fat (4 g sat); 6 g fiber; 37 g protein

Easy Saag Paneer

Prep 25 m
Total Time:25 m
4 servings

Ingredients

- ¾ teaspoon salt
- 1 small onion, finely chopped
- 1 jalapeño pepper, finely chopped (optional)
- 1 tspoon ground cumin
- 20 oz frozen spinach, thawed and finely chopped
- 1 clove garlic, minced
- 8 oz paneer cheese, cut into ½-inch cubes
- ¼ tspoon ground turmeric
- 2 tbspoons extra-virgin olive oil, divided
- 1 tbspoon minced fresh ginger
- 2 teaspoons garam masala
- 2 cups low-fat plain yogurt

Instructions

- In a medium bowl, mix the paneer with the turmeric until coated. Heat 1 spoonful of oil over medium heat in a large, non-stick skillet. Add the paneer and cook for about 5 minutes, flipping once, until both sides brown. Switch onto a platform.
- Adding the remaining 1 tablespoon of oil into the saucepan. Add the onion and jalapeño (if used) and cook, frequently stirring, for 7 to 8 minutes, until golden brown. (If the saucepan seems to be dry when cooking, add a little water, 2 tablespoons at a time.)

- Add garlic, ginger, masala garam, and cumin. Cook, stirring for about 30 seconds until it is fragrant. Season with spinach and oil.
- Cook for about 3 minutes, stirring, until dry. Remove from the heat and whisk in paneer and yogurt.

Nutrition Info

382 calories
24 g fat (12 g sat)
5 g fiber
19 g carbohydrates
25 g protein
223 mcg folate
64 mg cholesterol

Korean Grilled Mackerel

Active 30 m
Total Time:1 h
4 servings
Ingredients

- 2 tblespoons Korean chile paste
- 1 tblespoon canola oil
- 1 tblespoon reduced-sodium soy sauce
- 2 tspoons rice vinegar
- 1 tspoon grated fresh ginger
- 2 whole mackerel (about 1½ pounds each) or 4 whole rainbow trout (about 5 oz each), cleaned and butterflied, tails left on

Instructions

- In a small bowl, whisk chili paste, oil, soy sauce, vinegar, and ginger, until smooth. Move 2 spoonfuls of the marinade into a small bowl and set aside. Open every fish like a novel, and show the meat. Place the remaining marinade in a large saucepan or on a baking sheet over the meat. Marinate for 30 mins to 1 hour in the fridge. About 20 minutes before grilling, preheating the grill, or preparing a charcoal fire. Clean the grill rack, and oil well. Grill the fish for 3 minutes, flesh side down. Flip with a large spatula, spread the reserved marinade over the fish and grill until 3-4 minutes more opaque in the center.

Notes:

- You'll need whole mackerel (or rainbow trout) washed, butterflied, and the heads removed (tails left on) for this recycle. The availability of whole mackerel (or trout) varies, but most fish markets or fish departments will order and clean the fish for you at large supermarkets. Call forward to ensure you are getting what you're looking for.
- Korean chili paste (also known as hot pepper paste, gochujang or kochujang) is a fermented spicy condiment made with red chilies, soybeans, and salt. Order it on koamart.com or online in the Korean or Asian markets. Annie Chun, a widely distributed national Asian food brand, has recently launched its own bottled gochujang sauce, increasingly available in large supermarkets. It stays in the refrigerator forever. Combine 2 tablespoons of white miso, 2 tablespoons of Asian-style chili sauce, such as sriracha, and 2 teaspoons of molasses to make a substitute for Korean chili paste.

- Tip: Oil a grill rack, oil a folded paper towel, hold it over the rack with tongs and rub it. Fish on foil: Fish that flakes easily requires a delicate touch to flip on the grill. (Don't make use of a cooking spray on a hot grill) When grilling, if you want to miss turning it over, weigh a piece of foil large enough to hold the fish and cover it with a cooking spray. Grill the fish onto the foil (without turning) until it quickly flakes and reaches an inner temperature of 145°F.
- People having celiac disease or gluten sensitivity should use soy sauces that are labeled "gluten-free" because soy sauce that contains wheat or other sweeteners and flavors containing gluten.

Nutrition Info

221 calories; 7 g fat (1 g sat); 0 g fiber; 4 g carbohydrates; 34 g protein; 12 mcg folate; 87 mg cholesterol; 0 g sugars

Red Cabbage Salad and Blue Cheese with Maple-Glazed Walnuts

Active 35 m
Total Time: 35 m
8 servings

Ingredients

- 1 tablespoon crumbled blue cheese
- ¼ cup extra-virgin olive oil
- 3 tbspoons red-wine vinegar
- 1 tbspoon Dijon mustard
- ¼ tspoon salt
- ¼ tspoon freshly ground pepper
- 1 tblespoon extra-virgin olive oil
- 1 tspoon butter
- 1 cup walnuts
- ¼ tspoon salt
- ¼ tspoon freshly ground pepper
- 3 tblespoons pure maple syrup
- 8 cups very thinly sliced red cabbage
- 2 scallions, thinly sliced
- 1/4 cup crumbled blue cheese

Instructions

- To make the vinaigrette: in a mini food processor or blender, mix 1 tablespoon blue cheese, 1/4 cup butter, vinegar, mustard, salt, and pepper; process until creamy. Put/place a piece of parchment or wax paper near your stove to prepare the salad. Heat 1 spoonful of oil and butter over medium heat in a medium skillet.

- Attach the walnuts, and cook for 2 minutes, stirring. In maple syrup, add salt and pepper and drizzle. Cook, stirring, for 3 mins to 5 minutes until the nuts are well coated and have started to caramelize. Switch to paper, spooning over any remaining syrup.
- Separate the nuts while still moist. Let stand for about 5 minutes, until it is cold.
- Place the scallions and cabbage in a wide bowl. Place on the vinaigrette. Serve topped with walnuts and blue cheese.

Store airtight glazed walnuts (Step 2) to 1 day.

Nutrition info

19 g fat (4 g sat); 2 g fiber; 12 g carbohydrates; 232 calories; 4 g protein

Tips For The Anti-Inflammatory Diet.

Aging and inflammation go hand in hand as markers for inflammation-especially the ESR (erythrocyte sedimentation rate)-increase slowly with each decade. Most age-related illnesses have inflammation as their common denominator, and this is partly modulated by diet, so here are ten simple tips to prevent accumulation as much as possible of harmful inflammation products: skip the sugar. Diabetes is the basic model of accelerated aging, and anyway, sugar is made from empty calories. I know the desire to eat glucose is inherent but instead prefer fresh fruit salads. You'll be getting your sugar fix on the side and some nutrients.

- The sweet tooth is the reason that most people find it hard to lead a healthy lifestyle, and the majority of typical sweets are made of eggs, milk, butter, and flour baked in the oven. This is the perfect recipe for advanced end-products of glycation: you have protein, sugar, and high temperature. Maillard's reaction is the result. When time goes by, we're still' baking' from within, so why add more glycation? In return, you should try raw vegan desserts. These are made of nuts, seeds, and fruits and do not require heating or baking, which is why they are made faster. Hard vegan cake shops have begun springing up all over the place recently. If you do not live in such a place, search for raw vegan dessert recipes online, particularly if you have a weakness for sweets.

- Do not let a day pass without eating a salad and add as many fresh ingredients as possible to it.

- Evite smoked cheese and beef. The same is true for grilled meats. You have the miserable combination of high temperatures and proteins that quickly get denatured in both cases. Consumption of such product types is correlated with digestive cancers in populations where they are consumed in high quantities. There are safer ways to prepare foods for animals, so why risk it? You can try marinated fish or fermented cheese that is not smoked. Eat as few animal products as possible-this should suffice once a week.

- Use as low a cooking temperature as possible. If you're baking peppers, you might be able to use a lower temperature and a longer time than if you were baking beef. You wouldn't want to eat raw meats and get infections, of course. Just make the most of your best judgment while cooking.

- Use high levels of moisture when cooking. Boiling and broiling are way better than roasting or frying foods. That would be hard to implement if you're a lover of crispy foods. On the other hand, there are many fresh vegetables and fruits which, if you feel the need for it, are naturally crispy-peppers anybody?

- You don't need the cooking oil. A pot of ceramics and a little water will do, and food will not last. Afterwards, washing is a breeze.

- Evite heating up of fats. You can later also add cheese, avocado, nuts, and seeds to your recipes. Don't bake those, fry them, or roast them. If you put it over steamy fresh potatoes, the cheese will melt anyway, and the end result is just as good.

- Water should be your default beverage. Anything else-soups, teas, etc.-is a bonus, because it will never be replaced, even if the human body deals with what's available and removes energy from it. People get dehydrated with age anyway, and if you don't drink enough water, many substances precipitate, so why speed things up when water is so freely available and cheap? Unfortunately for everyone, this is not the case.

Eat as fresh as possible. If you want to eat meat or fish, get it fresh and use the frozen ingredients only if there is nothing else. Cook no more food than you eat in a single sitting. Heated food is not as fresh or tasty as one which is readily prepared. O late at this? I get it completely; this is why new vegetables, fruits, and nuts were first invented! If you do not have time to cook, you might add some quality yogurt and other healthy snacks.

Conclusion

Inflammation affects many aspects of our lives. It plays an essential part in our body, and we cannot do without it. But even as it protects us and plays a critical role in protecting us, if it gets out of control, there can be problems. They refer to it as chronic inflammation when this occurs.

It can seem a bit odd that something so important to our well-being and good health may also destroy our health and even cause death, but it is real. Chronic inflammation is certainly something you want to prevent.